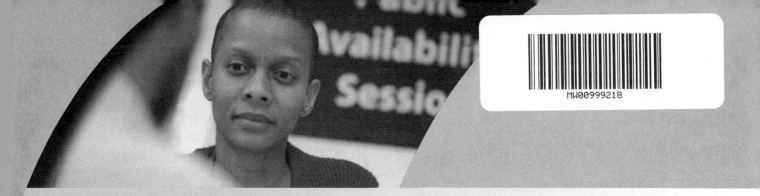

Essentials of Management and Leadership in Public Health

Robert E. Burke, PhD

Gordon A. Friesen Professor of Health Care Administration
School of Public Health and Health Services
The George Washington University
Washington, DC

Leonard H. Friedman, PhD, MPH

Professor
Department of Health Services Management and Leadership
School of Public Health and Health Services
The George Washington University
Washington, DC

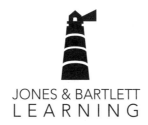

JONES & BARTLETT
LEARNING

World Headquarters
Jones & Bartlett Learning
5 Wall Street
Burlington, MA 01803
978-443-5000
info@jblearning.com
www.jblearning.com

Jones & Bartlett Learning books and products are available through most bookstores and online booksellers. To contact Jones & Bartlett Learning directly, call 800-832-0034, fax 978-443-8000, or visit our website, www.jblearning.com.

Substantial discounts on bulk quantities of Jones & Bartlett Learning publications are available to corporations, professional associations, and other qualified organizations. For details and specific discount information, contact the special sales department at Jones & Bartlett Learning via the above contact information or send an email to specialsales@jblearning.com.

This publication is designed to provide accurate and authoritative information in regard to the Subject Matter covered. It is sold with the understanding that the publisher is not engaged in rendering legal, accounting, or other professional service. If legal advice or other expert assistance is required, the service of a competent professional person should be sought.

Some images in this book feature models. These models do not necessarily endorse, represent, or participate in the activities represented in the images.

Production Credits
Publisher: Michael Brown
Editorial Assistant: Catie Heverling
Editorial Assistant: Teresa Reilly
Production Manager: Tracey Chapman
Senior Marketing Manager: Sophie Fleck
Manufacturing and Inventory Control Supervisor: Amy Bacus
Composition: Auburn Associates, Inc.
Image Credit: © AbleStock
Cover Design: Kristin E. Parker
Cover Image: Top left: © CDC/Dawn Arlotta; Top right: © CDC/Dawn Arlotta; Bottom: Photo credit: James Gathany, Centers for Disease Control and Prevention
Printing and Binding: Edwards Brothers Malloy
Cover Printing: Edwards Brothers Malloy

Library of Congress Cataloging-in-Publication Data
Burke, Robert E.
  Essentials of management and leadership in public health / Robert E. Burke, Leonard H. Friedman.
     p. ; cm.
  Includes bibliographical references and index.
  ISBN-13: 978-0-7637-4291-1 (pbk.)
  ISBN-10: 0-7637-4291-0 (pbk.)
  1. Health services administration. I. Friedman, Leonard H. II. Title.
  [DNLM: 1. Public Health Administration—methods. 2. Personnel Management—methods. 3. Public Health Practice.
WA 525 B959e 2010]
  RA971.B895 2010
  362.1068—dc22
                                                              2010000294
6048
Printed in the United States of America
17 16 15 14   10 9 8 7 6 5 4

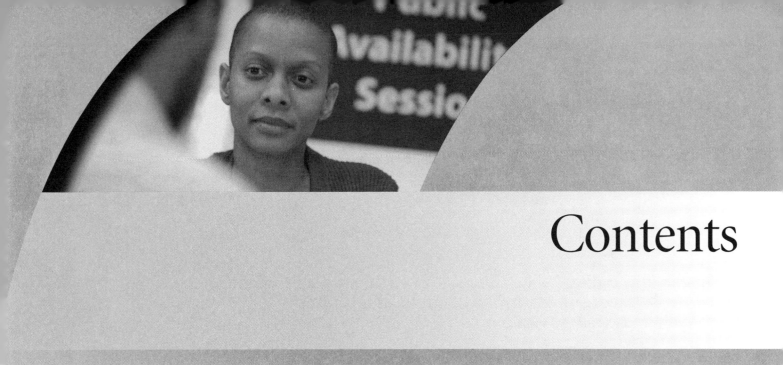

Contents

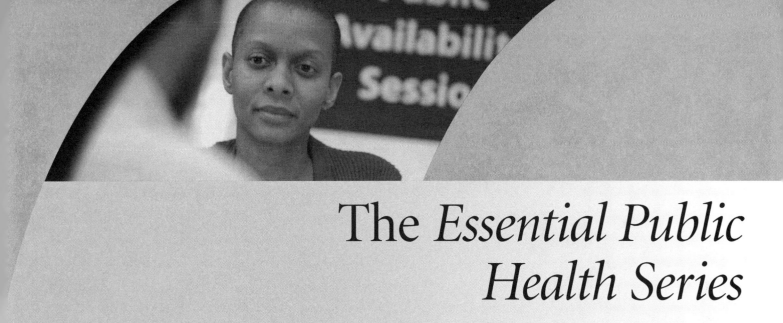

The *Essential Public Health Series*

Log on to www.essentialpublichealth.com *for the most current information on availability.*

CURRENT AND FORTHCOMING TITLES IN THE *ESSENTIAL PUBLIC HEALTH SERIES*:

Public Health 101: Healthy People–Healthy Populations—Richard Riegelman, MD, MPH, PhD

Essentials of Public Health—Bernard J. Turnock, MD, MPH

Essential Case Studies in Public Health: Putting Public Health into Practice—Katherine Hunting, PhD, MPH &
   Brenda L. Gleason, MA, MPH

Essentials of Evidence-Based Public Health—Richard Riegelman, MD, MPH, PhD

Epidemiology 101—Robert H. Friis, PhD

Essentials of Infectious Disease Epidemiology—Manya Magnus, PhD, MPH

Essential Readings in Infectious Disease Epidemiology—Manya Magnus, PhD, MPH

Essentials of Biostatistics in Public Health—Lisa M. Sullivan, PhD (with Workbook: Statistical Computations Using Excel)

Essentials of Public Health Biology: A Guide for the Study of Pathophysiology—Constance Urciolo Battle, MD

Essentials of Environmental Health—Robert H. Friis, PhD

Essentials of Global Health—Richard Skolnik, MPA

Case Studies in Global Health: Millions Saved—Ruth Levine, PhD & the What Works Working Group

Essentials of Health, Culture, and Diversity—Mark Edberg, PhD

Essentials of Health Behavior: Social and Behavioral Theory in Public Health—Mark Edberg, PhD

Essential Readings in Health Behavior: Theory and Practice—Mark Edberg, PhD

Essentials of Health Policy and Law—Joel B. Teitelbaum, JD, LLM & Sara E. Wilensky, JD, MPP

Essential Readings in Health Policy and Law—Joel B. Teitelbaum, JD, LLM & Sara E. Wilensky, JD, MPP

Essentials of Health Economics—Diane M. Dewar, PhD

Essentials of Global Community Health—Jaime Gofin, MD, MPH & Rosa Gofin, MD, MPH

Essentials of Program Planning and Evaluation—Karen McDonnell, PhD

Essentials of Public Health Communication—Claudia Parvanta, PhD; Patrick Remington, MD, MPH; Ross Brownson, PhD;
   & David E. Nelson, MD, MPH

Essentials of Public Health Ethics—Ruth Gaare Bernheim, JD, MPH & James F. Childress, PhD

Essentials of Management and Leadership in Public Health—Robert Burke, PhD & Leonard Friedman, PhD, MPH

Essentials of Public Health Preparedness—Rebecca Katz, PhD, MPH

ABOUT THE EDITOR:

Richard K. Riegelman, MD, MPH, PhD, is Professor of Epidemiology-Biostatistics, Medicine, and Health Policy, and Founding Dean of The George Washington University School of Public Health and Health Services in Washington, DC. He has taken a lead role in developing the Educated Citizen and Public Health initiative which has brought together arts and sciences and public health education associations to implement the Institute of Medicine of the National Academies' recommendation that "…all undergraduates should have access to education in public health." Dr. Riegelman also led the development of George Washington's undergraduate major and minor and currently teaches "Public Health 101" and "Epidemiology 101" to undergraduates.

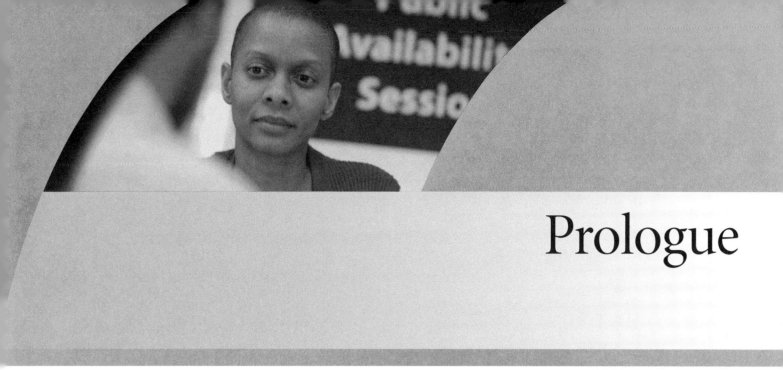

Prologue

Understanding the foundations of management is not just for managers. Appreciating the roles that management plays in getting the work of the world done is critical for all those who seek to understand public health.

Public health requires the full range of management skills—from budgeting to personnel, from planning to marketing. It also requires the personal skills of leadership that are so essential to the success of public health organizations. *Essentials of Management and Leadership in Public Health* provides insight into these diverse aspects of management and links them to the roles they play in public health.

Having completed the book, students will not be ready to manage but rather to appreciate what good managers and leaders do and how they do it. Thus, *Essentials of Management and Leadership in Public Health* is a good place to begin if your goal is to become a manager or to work with managers, which pretty much means all of us, regardless of our chosen field.

The roles of management are addressed through the perspective of leadership. Leadership is indispensable to the success of organizations over the long run. Understanding how the day-to-day roles of management relate to leadership is to understand the big picture of what management needs to do to succeed.

As the editors recognize, management can be thought of as a fundamental cross-cutting discipline, drawing on a wide range of specific fields of study. Therefore, the editors have brought together a highly experienced group of authors from a wide range of disciplines.

Essentials of Management and Leadership in Public Health's authors are also experienced managers. They share the common link of teaching in the Department of Health Services Management and Leadership of The George Washington University School of Public Health and Health Services, which is chaired by Robert Burke. Leonard Friedman and Robert Burke have worked hard to provide the book with a common voice and coherent approach.

Essentials of Management and Leadership in Public Health is central to the understanding of public health and the role it plays in protecting and promoting health and minimizing disease and disabilities. I am pleased that *Essentials of Management and Leadership* is a part of our *Essential Public Health Series*. It is an important book—whether you are new to public health or are reviewing basic principles in preparation for the certifying examination. Take a careful look, and you will take away concepts that will serve you well for many years to come.

Richard K. Riegelman MD, MPH, PhD
Editor, *Essential Public Health Series*

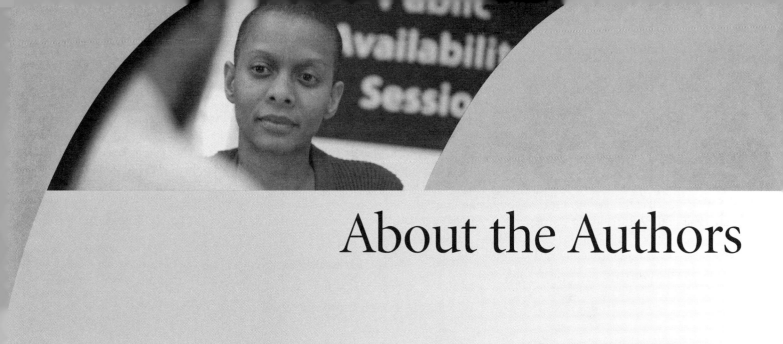

About the Authors

Robert E. Burke, PhD

Robert E. Burke is the Gordon A. Friesen Professor of Health Care Administration and Chair of the Department of Health Services Management and Leadership. He teaches courses in long-term care management, global health management, health behavior, and advocacy. He holds joint appointments in the Department of Health Policy and the Program in Health Sciences. In 2008, the Secretary of the Department of Veterans Affairs appointed Dr. Burke to a congressionally mandated Veterans Committee on Disability Determination that was an outgrowth of the Dole Shalala Commission.

Professor Burke is a medical sociologist and a nationally known expert in long-term care, with extensive experience in developing, evaluating, and implementing healthcare policy and managing multidisciplinary professional staff. He has conducted and directed health service research, payment, and evaluation projects, and is thoroughly versed in the policy and program issues of Medicare, Medicaid, and other public and private third-party payer systems.

As Department Chair, Professor Burke oversees a well-known and well-respected faculty that has been in continuous existence for fifty years. Dr. Burke held senior research positions at the Institute of Medicine, the General Accounting Office (now the Government Accountability Office), the Health and Retirement Funds of the United Mine Workers, and the Pepper Commission. He has worked with the Health Care Financing Administration (now The Centers for Medicare and Medicaid Services), directing the design of prospective payments systems for post-acute care.

Education

Master of Arts (Sociology), Boston College, 1970
Doctor of Philosophy (Medical Sociology), University of Florida, 1977

Leonard H. Friedman, PhD, MPH

Leonard H. Friedman is a Professor in the Department of Health Services Management and Leadership, and Director of the Master of Health Services Administration program. Dr. Friedman also holds a faculty appointment in the Department of Health Policy.

Dr. Leonard Friedman is an expert on the mechanisms of organizational change and strategic decision-making in health service organizations. He joined SPHHS in 2008 from Oregon State University, where he was professor in the Department of Public Health and coordinator of the school's health management and policy programs.

In his years in academia, Dr. Friedman's scholarly interests have evolved from the mechanisms by which hospitals decide to adopt certain technological innovations in clinical settings, to the underperformance of integrated health systems, to developing a model of organizational change practices. Dr. Friedman's research interests in health care management centers around strategic management, organizational theory and behavior, and decision making in complex and uncertain environments.

Professor Friedman has taught classes in healthcare management, organizational theory and behavior in health care, healthcare law and regulation, and strategic management and leadership in healthcare organizations. As part of his dedication to the field, Dr. Friedman has chaired the Health Care Management Division of the Academy of Management and is a member of the governing council at the Institute for Healthcare Improvement's Health Professions Education Collaborative. He has also been board chair of the Association of University Programs in Health Administration.

He received both his Bachelor of Arts degree and his Master of Public Health degree from California State University, Northridge. He was awarded both his Master of Public Administration degree and a Doctor of Philosophy in Public Administration from the University of Southern California, 1991.

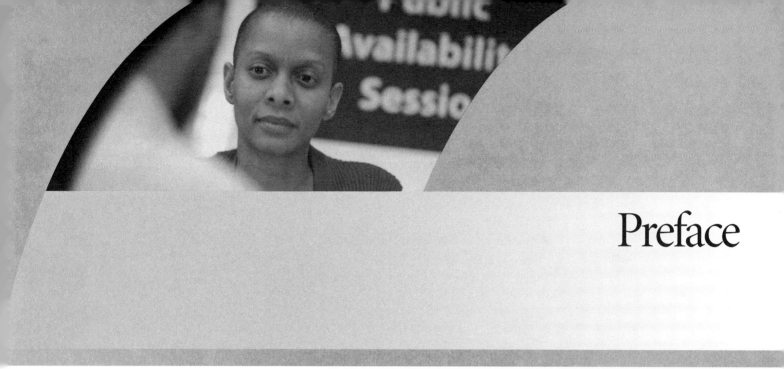

Preface

This book is a composite of the best ideas and concepts garnered from the various specialties that comprise management and leadership in public health. The editors of this text posit that it takes many hands, skills, and talents to enable a person to evolve into an effective and respected leader and manager. As such, the editors sought authors who shared this perspective and invited these area experts to be chapter authors. The breadth of topics and expertise of the authors clearly exemplify the ideals and purpose of this book. The topics and writers also reflect the diversity and training of the faculty of our department of health services management and leadership. Taken as a whole, these various specialties and professionals come together such that "WE ARE ALL PUBLIC HEALTH MANAGEMENT."

Peter Drucker was for many people the best-known and most highly respected management thinker of the 20th century. In 1989, writing in the Harvard Business Review, he observed: "Nonprofits need management even more than business does, precisely because they lack the discipline of the bottom line." This implied focus on an organization's desire to improve the human condition suggests a lack of concern with profitability and economic stability that directs publicly traded corporations. We believe that Professor Drucker would have applied the same logic to public health organizations. This is the objective of this book—to provide the readers with the information and perspective needed to become exceptional managers and leaders. Public health organizations include (but are not limited to) county and state health departments, community service agencies, and other nongovernmental organizations. All of these require managers who possess the skill and ability to guide the highly trained professional staff, support personnel, and generous volunteers through turbulent and uncertain environments.

Public health organizations are similar to their counterparts in the private sector where staff members who are very successful at the jobs for which they have specifically been educated are frequently recognized for their good work by being promoted into a management role. The assumption is that persons who are successful in the job for which they were originally hired will be equally successful in managing and leading others. We note an incongruity here that seems to permeate virtually every organizational form. While formal education (and even licensure) is needed for most public health jobs, management roles require nothing other than common sense, familiarity with the organization's policies and procedures manual, an orientation to specific rules and regulations, and in certain enlightened organizations, an off-site weekend-long intensive seminar on personnel management. We believe the idea that management requires no particular education, preparation, or talent is at best naïve and at worst dangerous to the health and well-being of the organization and the clients served.

We have worked to craft a textbook in management and leadership in public health with one assumption and two goals in mind. Our assumption is that management and leadership are two sides of the same coin. Both activities are action oriented and are ultimately about getting things done. The difference is perspective. We concur that Warren Bennis was right when he said that managers do things right and leaders do the right things (Bennis and Nanus, 1985).

The first of our goals is to give the readers the basic tools they will need to become effective managers and leaders in their organization. There are a set of theories and skills that come together to form the foundation of the tool kit of management and leadership. This book explicitly sets out to help new managers identify the important tools they will need in this role, or in the case of more experienced managers, develop their abilities to better use those tools. The second goal of this book is to help light a spark in the reader to learn more about management and leadership. One book, no matter how well-written, is a necessary but not sufficient condition. There is so much more that can be read and learned. In fact, universities have courses as well as undergraduate and graduate degree programs dedicated to management and leadership. We hope that you will take this book as the first step in your journey to develop a deeper and more profound understanding of the many talents and skills management and leadership require.

One final thought cycles back to our assumption about management and leadership. Reading about this is not enough. Getting better in these roles requires you to actually get out and participate in managerial and leadership roles. In this way, you will know whether you have the innate talent and ability to be truly successful as a manager and leader. Communities around the world depend on well-managed and skillfully led public health organizations to provide needed services in a safe, efficient, and effective manner. We appreciate your taking the first step on this important journey. We encourage your diligence and, most importantly, we look forward to being witnesses to your success at leading and managing public health programs and services in the years ahead.

Robert E. Burke, PhD
Leonard H. Friedman, PhD, MPH
Co-editors

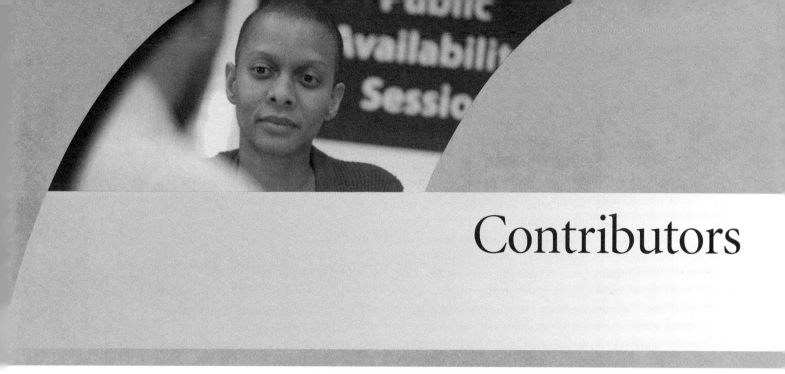

Contributors

Douglas Anderson, MHA, FACMPE

Beginning in 2004, Mr. Anderson has been a faculty member in the Department of Health Services Management and Leadership in the School of Public Health and Health Services at The George Washington University. His teaching responsibilities include Physician Practice Management, Introduction to Economics and Management Principles in Healthcare, and Healthcare Policy Analysis.

For the past 30 years, Professor Anderson successfully managed and directed physician group medical practices and has written and presented in this area of health policy. His work experience includes functioning as the Chief Executive Officer of a multi-site orthopaedic group practice, the CEO of a multi-site, multi-state ophthalmology group practice, the Chief Operating Officer of a multi-state, multi-specialty medical group practice, and the COO of a multi-site primary care practice. He also established a Medical Services Organization for an integrated health delivery system operating in a three-state region, and provided development resources to affiliated medical practices and individual physicians.

Professor Anderson provides consultative services to medical groups, and is an active member in the Medical Group Management Association. A respected and gifted speaker, he is known for giving presentations on medical practice management at the local, state, and national level. He achieved life member status as a Fellow in the American College of Medical Practice Executives.

Professor Anderson has a BA in Psychology from the University of North Carolina at Chapel Hill and a Masters in Health Administration from Duke University. At this time, he is pursuing a PhD in Public Policy from George Mason University, with a concentration in health policy. His research interests focus on the policy implications of the organizational structure of medical group practice organizations.

Philip Aspden, MA, PhD

Philip Aspden has consulted in telecommunications and technology-based economic development for a wide range of high-tech firms, public bodies, and foundations, both in the United States and Europe. Earlier, he was a scientific civil servant in the British Civil Service and a research scholar at the International Institute for Applied Systems Analysis, Vienna, Austria. Dr. Aspden is a Senior Program Officer on the staff of the Board on Science, Technology, and Economic Policy at the National Academy of Sciences.

Kurt J. Darr, JD, ScD

Kurt J. Darr is a Professor of Hospital Administration in the Department of Health Services Management and Leadership. Dr. Darr's main research interests center on health services ethics, hospital and medical staff organization and management, quality and productivity improvements, and applying the Deming method in health services delivery.

It is the "ah-ha" moment on the face of a student who suddenly grasps a complex concept that helps Dr. Darr feel so professionally fulfilled. Since his first full-time academic appointment at The George Washington University in 1973, he has found the elusive "joy in work," a concept described by the master management theorist W. Edwards Deming.

Dr. Darr gained hands-on experience as an administrator at the Mayo Clinic and in the US Navy Medical Service Corps before turning to a career in academics. In addition to a doctoral degree, he has completed post-doctoral fellowships with the Department of Health, Education, and Welfare (now the Department of Health and Human Services), the World Health Organization, and what is now the Commission on Accreditation of Healthcare Management Education.

He received his Bachelor of Arts in History and Political Science at Concordia College, both his Juris Doctor and his Master of Hospital Administration at The University of Minnesota School of Law, and was awarded his Doctor of Science from The Johns Hopkins University School of Hygiene and Public Health.

Steven R. Eastaugh, ScD

Steven R. Eastaugh is a Professor in the Department of Health Services Management and Leadership. Dr. Eastaugh's main research interests include health finance and economics, capital budgeting, financial ratio analysis, profitability and liquidity, cost-benefit and cost-effectiveness, and technology assessment. For the past thirty years, Dr. Eastaugh has taught health finance and economics. The author of seven books and more than 140 journal articles, Dr. Eastaugh is a nationally acclaimed speaker, consultant, and agent of change who has traveled to some 36 countries as part of his health services research.

Prior to coming to The George Washington University, Dr. Eastaugh taught at Cornell University and was a senior staff health economist at the National Academy of Sciences. He was trained at both Harvard and The Johns Hopkins Universities, where he received his Bachelor of Arts in Biochemistry and Economics, Master of Science in Public Health, Harvard University, and Doctor of Science in Public Health, Johns Hopkins School of Hygiene and Public Health.

Pamela Clapp Larmee, CFRE

Pamela Clapp Larmee, CFRE has over fifteen years of fundraising experience focused in higher education and health care. She is an independent consultant providing fundraising and strategic planning services including program development, board leadership, volunteer management, and campaign strategy. She has worked with John Wm. Thomas Consulting, LLC and Capital Development Strategies for clients including the National Health Museum, the International Society for Quality of Life Research, and the National Association of Criminal Defense Lawyers.

Pam is the former Associate Vice President of Medical Center Advancement at The George Washington University in Washington, DC. For five years, she led the overall development and alumni relations efforts of the Medical Center, including the School of Medicine and Health Sciences and the School of Public Health and Health Services. She also was responsible for the creation and implementation of a grateful patient fundraising program. She holds an English degree from the University of Michigan and an Association for Healthcare Philanthropy (AHP) certificate in fundraising management.

Blaine Parrish, PhD, MA

Blaine Parrish is Associate Dean for Student Affairs and Assistant Professor in the Department of Health Policy. For the School of Public Health and Health Services (SPHHS) he teaches courses in Management Approaches to Public Health, and for the Department of Health Policy he teaches Advanced Health Policy Analysis.

An expert in the field of leadership, organization, and management, Dr. Parrish's scholarly interests focus on community-based organizations that provide public health services to vulnerable and underserved populations. He joined SPHHS in 2002 as program manager at the Forum for Collaborative HIV Research, which is affiliated with the Department of Prevention and Community Health. The Forum is a public-private partnership that facilitates discussion on emerging issues in HIV clinical research and works to transfer research results into care. In earlier positions, Dr. Parrish served as a public health analyst in the HIV/AIDS Bureau at the Health Resources and Services Administration (HRSA).

Dr. Parrish earned his Bachelor of Arts at the University of Central Oklahoma, his Master of Arts at the University of Texas at Arlington, and was awarded his Doctor of Philosophy at Cappella University.

Sara Rosenbaum, JD

Sara Rosenbaum is Chair of the Department of Health Policy and Harold and Jane Hirsh Professor of Health Law and Policy. She also holds an appointment as Professor of Health Care Sciences at The George Washington University's School of Medicine and Law.

As a scholar, educator, and national leader, Professor Rosenbaum has dedicated her career to promoting more equitable and effective healthcare policies in this country, particularly in the areas of Medicaid and Medicare, managed care, employee health benefits, maternal and child health, community health centers, and civil rights in healthcare systems. Her commitment to strengthening access to care for low-income, minority, and medically underserved populations has had a transforming effect on the lives of many Americans, particularly children.

Professor Rosenbaum's research focuses on the many ways in which the law intersects with the nation's healthcare and public health systems, with a particular emphasis on civil rights, quality of care, insurance coverage, and managed care. She is co-author of *Law and the American Health Care System*, a widely used health law textbook.

As a noted scholar, public officials, the media, and healthcare organizations regularly seek Professor Rosenbaum's expertise. She serves on the board of numerous national organizations.

Ms. Rosenbaum received her Bachelor of Arts from Wesleyan University and her Juris Doctor from Boston University School of Law.

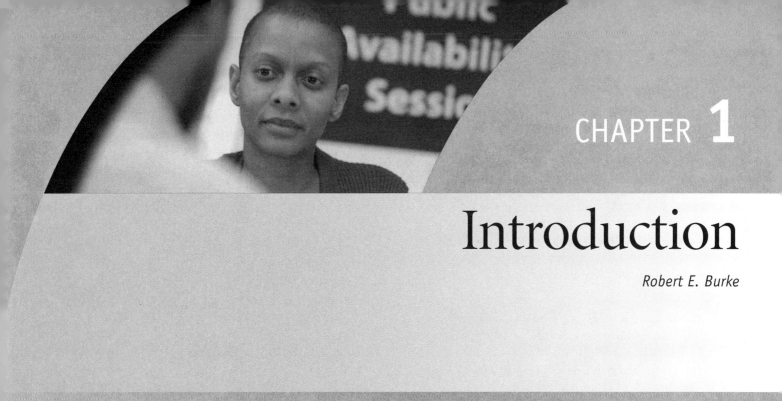

CHAPTER 1

Introduction

Robert E. Burke

For the student pursuing studies in public health, the role of management and the reason for studying management is unclear if not counterintuitive. It is one of the many goals for this text that students who study public health management will obtain the insight that management principles apply to all aspects of human endeavor. While it is leadership that creates the vision, it is management that makes the vision happen. For reasons that baffle the authors of this text, there are people who dedicate themselves to the "greater good" (including public health), but misunderstand management and the need for using tested and valid management principles. To these uninformed, management is seen negatively. It is perceived only as a way in which corporations use some magic models of efficiency that result in increased productivity and greater profit for investors. Some believe that management has no benefit for the recipients of public health programs nor for the professionals who staff these programs. It has been the authors' experience that many public health students want to finish their public health education and then obtain critical public health jobs as soon as they have completed their bachelor's or master's degrees (if not sooner). These public health workers are eager to be the next epidemiologist; to work to test the quality of air and water; or to design, implement, and evaluate the next health education programs that will better the outcomes of a population. Public health students want to enter the job force to create better, more comprehensive health promotion and health awareness programs. They are eager to become the next talented community health professionals who are advocates for population-based medicine. These are all noble goals, but they are not complete. What is missing are knowledge, understanding, and application of public health management.

It is the contention of the editors and authors of this text, however, that management—good management—is integral to all public health activities, and without management, public health activities are far less effective and may even be impossible. The authors further contend that many times management courses as taught in schools of public health are aimed at teaching how to operate and manage the day-to-day operations of a public health program. These may be strong practical courses, but they do not provide an overall management perspective, nor do they demonstrate how leadership will enable the public health professional to ensure that public health goals and objectives are successfully achieved. As such, the student never understands the importance of management in and of itself and how this noble academic pursuit fits into the world of public health. This is the goal of this text.

WHY STUDY MANAGEMENT?

From the time the editors and authors envisioned this text, its goals, the format, and the topics addressed, to the time when the authors began to write, the content has changed to meet the changing needs of population health management. The editors chose not to look at the management of specific public health programs but instead to use these programs to exemplify and clarify a management construct, idea, or theory. Based on the authors' distinct and different academic backgrounds, the editors realized that many public health workers learn management skills as an add-on to their public health training and not as an integral part of their education. Some public health students learn management concepts after they receive their master's of public health (MPH) degree; some learn management skills "on-the-job"; while some never really learn, grasp, or value management as an integral skill. As presented in this text, management is shown to be a compilation of many different disciplines and skill sets. This book demonstrates that no one academic discipline holds the market on management as a legitimate academic pursuit. The authors define *management* in this book in the following ways:

- It is first and foremost an interdisciplinary, rigorous, and valid endeavor that is integral to all human enterprise, including public health.
- It is both a necessary and sufficient condition to ensure the goals of public health programs are met.
- It is an integral component of the social contract.

These ideas and concepts of the authors of this text have been validated by the Council on Education for Public Health (CEPH). CEPH has expressed the importance of management to public health, and has determined that management, as a component of health policy and management, is one of the

five core competencies areas for public health. The management competencies that a public health professional must have are listed in **Tables 1-1** and **1-2**.

Except for the policy competencies (D.3 and D.4), each of these competencies is addressed. The leadership cross-cutting competencies are also contained throughout the different chapters in this book.

WHAT IS MANAGEMENT?

The authors of this text all share the view that management is not one concept or idea. Good management as practiced by public health professionals is a compilation of concepts from many different professions and professionals. In fact, management could be considered one of the first cross-cutting academic disciplines. As presented in this text, management ideas, thought development, and action are steeped in sociology, psychology, social psychology, behavioral sciences, economics, management theory, statistics, and finance.

The authors of this text represent these disciplines and share the beliefs that all management is cross-cutting and that management is a necessary correlate of and for public health. Each of the authors is an experienced manager in the private and/or public sector. Each has received education and training

---

TABLE 1-1 Management Competencies, Health Policy and Management

D. Health Policy and Management[*]

Health policy and management is a multidisciplinary field of inquiry and practice concerned with the delivery, quality, and costs of health care for individuals and populations. This definition assumes both a managerial and a policy concern with the structure, process, and outcomes of health services including the costs, financing, organization, outcomes, and accessibility of care.

Competencies: Upon graduation, a student with an MPH should be able to…

D.1 Identify the main components and issues of the organization, financing, and delivery of health services and public health systems in the United States.
D.2 Describe the legal and ethical bases for public health and health services.
D.3 Explain methods of ensuring community health safety and preparedness.
D.4 Discuss the policy process for improving the health status of populations.
D.5 Apply the principles of program planning, development, budgeting, management, and evaluation in organizational and community initiatives.
D.6 Apply principles of strategic planning and marketing to public health.
D.7 Apply quality and performance improvement concepts to address organizational performance issues.
D.8 Apply "systems thinking" for resolving organizational problems.
D.9 Communicate health policy and management issues using appropriate channels and technologies.
D.10 Demonstrate leadership skills for building partnerships.

[*]In this series, *health policy* is treated as a separate text and area of inquiry. As such, this text addresses only the health management competencies.
Source: ASPH.

TABLE 1-2 Management Competencies, Leadership

H. Leadership

The ability to create and communicate a shared vision for a changing future, champion solutions to organizational and community challenges, and energize commitment to goals.

Competencies: Upon graduation, it is increasingly important that a student with an MPH be able to...
H.1   Describe the attributes of leadership in public health.
H.2   Describe alternative strategies for collaboration and partnership among organizations, focused on public health goals.
H.3   Articulate an achievable mission, set of core values, and vision.
H.4   Engage in dialogue and learning from others to advance public health goals.
H.5   Demonstrate team building, negotiation, and conflict management skills.
H.6   Demonstrate transparency, integrity, and honesty in all actions.
H.7   Use collaborative methods for achieving organizational and community health goals.
H.8   Apply social justice and human rights principles when addressing community needs.
H.9   Develop strategies to motivate others for collaborative problem solving, decision making, and evaluation.

Source: ASPH.

---

in management, but the authors have different academic backgrounds. The authors include a medical sociologist, an economist, attorneys, health systems managers, a fund-raising specialist, a health services researcher, and a health systems information specialist. These authors are all "doers." In addition to academic appointments, they have held senior health services management jobs in the public and private sectors. Each is unique in the contribution he or she is making to public health management.

The primary goal of this text is to harness the public health manament experience of the authors so that this book is replete with several different and, at times, unique management perspectives. The student should learn that good management involves the implementation of problem-solving methods that may vary with each and every program, process, or situation. Because all public health is done with teamwork, the secondary goal is to teach future managers that to successfully write and co-author a chapter or paper, interdisciplinary teamwork is both desired and needed. This blending of ideas and backgrounds adds to the richness of the ideas and thoughts.

The third goal of this book is to present the value that all good efforts need to be successfully managed and that public health is no different. Working with the management ideas and perspectives presented in this book will enable public health professionals to more efficiently and effectively carry out the vision and mission of public health, which are defined by the American Public Health Association as follows:

Vision: *Healthy People in Healthy Communities*
Mission: *Promote Physical and Mental Health and Prevent Disease, Injury, and Disability*

PUBLIC HEALTH

- Prevents epidemics and the spread of disease.
- Protects against environmental hazards.
- Prevents injuries.
- Promotes and encourages healthy behaviors.
- Responds to disasters and assists communities in recovery.
- Ensures the quality and accessibility of health services.

ESSENTIAL PUBLIC HEALTH SERVICES

- Monitor health status to identify community health problems.
- Diagnose and investigate health problems and health hazards in the community.
- Inform, educate, and empower people about health issues.
- Mobilize community partnerships to identify and solve health problems.
- Develop policies and plans that support individual and community health efforts.
- Enforce laws and regulations that protect health and ensure safety.

- Link people to needed personal health services and ensure the provision of health care when otherwise unavailable.
- Ensure a competent public health and personal healthcare workforce.
- Evaluate effectiveness, accessibility, and quality of personal and population-based health services.
- Develop new insights and innovative solutions to health problems.

As **Figure 1-1** shows, the inner core connecting all the functions of public health is systems management. Management is the operational glue that keeps all components of public health together and enables its workers to meet the vision and mission of public health.

FRAMEWORK FOR THE BOOK AND THE STUDY OF MANAGEMENT

The authors posit that the study of management can be divided into three major areas:

1. Basic management theory.
2. Technology, including finance, economics, and information systems.
3. Advanced management skills.

The first area, basic management theory, is discussed here in Chapter 1, "Introduction," Chapter 2, "Introduction to Management and Leadership Concepts, Principles, and Practices," Chapter 4, "Strategic Planning and Marketing for Public Health Managers," and Chapter 9, "Managing Rela-

FIGURE 1-1

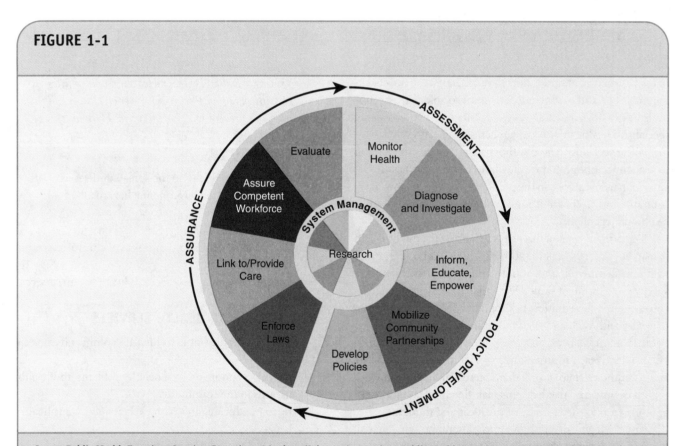

Source: Public Health Functions Steering Committee, Members (July 1995): American Public Health Association·Association of Schools of Public Health·Association of State and Territorial Health Officials·Environmental Council of the States·National Association of County and City Health Officials·National Association of State Alcohol and Drug Abuse Directors·National Association of State Mental Health Program Directors·Public Health Foundation·U.S. Public Health Service·Agency for Health Care Policy and Research·Centers for Disease Control and Prevention·Food and Drug Administration·Health Resources and Services Administration·Indian Health Service·National Institutes of Health·Office of the Assistant Secretary for Health·Substance Abuse and Mental Health Services Administration.

tionships and Effective Communication." The second area, technology, is discussed in Chapter 6, "Finance and Economics," Chapter 8, "Informatics in Public Health Management," and Chapter 11, "Fundraising, Grant Writing, Budgeting, and Project Management." The third area, advanced management skills, is addressed in Chapter 3, "Leading Public Health Organizations: Team Building, Reorganization, and Board Relationships," Chapter 5, "Conflict Resolution and Negotiation in Healthcare Management," Chapter 7, "Ethics and Professionalism in Public Health," Chapter 10, "Managing Complex and Culturally Diverse Workplaces," and Chapter 12, "Changing Role of Public Health Managers and Leaders."

Basic management chapters teach the public health student the "whys and wherefores" of management as it relates to public health. The technology chapters provide the public health manager with the practical and applied skills necessary for effective management. The advanced management skills chapters amalgamate and use the knowledge learned in the basic management and technology chapters to provide the public health manager with the tools to manage, lead, and address the complex areas that are crucial for today's public health manager. Ethics, leadership, law, diversity, and negotiation are the topics that frame the advanced management skills section.

The learning framework used in the book is a classic three-legged approach: theory, application, and practice. Generally, each chapter starts with the theoretical and historical underpinnings of the topic. Definitions and perspectives of the concept are presented. Applications of the topic to public health programs and public health management follow. Each chapter ends with discussion questions to augment the concepts.

Finally, it is the expectation of the authors that the students who read this book and who study public health management will become the next generation of leaders and managers. They will understand the need for managing population medicine in addition to individual medicine. These educated leaders will meet the challenges for public health in the 21st century. The first challenge is to lead the healthcare community of providers and clients to realize that effective management of community public health issues such as pandemics, flu, AIDS, obesity, and chronic disease, as well as health promotion and prevention, communication, epidemiology, environmental health, and occupational health and exercise, is the only effective way to ensure a nation and a future population of healthy people who can contribute to the continuing and future success of the country.

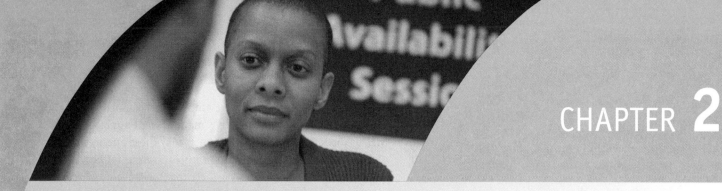

CHAPTER **2**

Introduction to Management and Leadership Concepts, Principles, and Practices

Kurt Darr

INTRODUCTION

Everyone manages. We manage our finances, time, careers, and relationships. We tend not to think of these activities as "managing" or of ourselves as being "managers." Nevertheless, they are. These examples of managing or being managers are relatively simple and straightforward, even though we may find many of them fraught with difficulty. It is when the concepts of managing or being a manager are applied to organizations that complexity increases—almost always exponentially. At this point it becomes necessary to study and understand the theoretical bases of management.

The practice of management and the classical enunciation of management principles can be traced to the 19th century. The development of management as an academic discipline based on a body of knowledge that can be taught is a recent development and is generally attributed to the work of Peter F. Drucker in the latter half of the 20th century. That body of knowledge is taught in graduate schools of business and in programs that prepare managers of public health departments, programs, and health services organizations, such as hospitals, clinics, and long-term care facilities. This chapter provides a basic introduction to management theory and problem solving, and concludes with a brief discussion of negotiation and alternative dispute resolution.

Managers are persons who are formally appointed to positions of authority in organizations. They enable others to do their work and are accountable to a higher authority for work results. Primarily, the differences between levels of managers are the degree of authority and the scope of their accountabil-

ity for work results. Line managers manage people and things; staff managers, such as the human resources department and the fiscal office, support the work of line managers.

LEARNING OBJECTIVES

After reading the chapter, the reader will be able to:

1. Review the background on managing and management.
2. Discuss organizational culture, philosophy, and performance.
3. Describe the elements of management knowledge.
4. Describe the five functions of management and decision making.
5. Discuss the distinctions between managing and leading.
6. Outline management skills, roles, and competencies.
7. Review the steps in managerial problem solving.
8. Discuss designing formal organizations.
9. Describe the contributions of contemporary management theorists.
10. Discuss negotiating and alternative dispute resolution.

ORGANIZATIONAL CULTURE, PHILOSOPHY, AND PERFORMANCE

Management, organization, culture, and organizational philosophy are inextricably linked; they are especially linked to organizational effectiveness. Much has been written about an organization's culture and the need for managers to not only understand the values in that culture, but to move that culture in the direction of values that further the organization's mission and vision. The value system of an organization can also be called its *organizational philosophy*—the ethical context in which goods and services are rendered. Ethics audits are an important tool managers can use to "biopsy" the organization's value system. These audits are comprised of staff surveys; observations of staff/patient interaction; and reviews of staff recruitment, selection, and training. Audits provide an understanding of the culture so that the culture's values can be moved in the desired direction.

Managers are judged by their organizations' performance. The way managers set standards, coordinate and integrate workgroups, make decisions, and design the organization affect performance. In addition, it is patently clear from research and anecdotal evidence that high-performing organizations have a values system that furthers the organization's goals. These values are expressed in explicit and implicit ways by managers and are expected to be present in the work of all members of the staff. Managers must model appropriate behavior. It is logical to conclude that an organization in which all staff understand the desired values and incorporate them into their work lives will achieve its goals more effectively.

MANAGEMENT THEORY

Management or managing has four main elements. It is (1) a process comprised of interrelated social and technical functions and activities (2) that accomplishes organizational objectives, (3) achieves these objectives through use of people and other resources, and (4) does so in a formal organizational setting. In concert with managers at various levels, senior management establishes organizational objectives, and all who work in the organization strive to achieve them. Management's work includes providing an organizational context in which direct and support work can be performed effectively, and preparing an organization to deal with threats and opportunities in its external environment.

Managers at all levels shape organizational values and culture by their decisions and through leading by example (modeling), even though senior managers usually have the clearest and most direct effect. The organization's overall performance is the best evidence of managers' efforts. Regardless of hierarchical level, managers throughout an organization engage in the same basic, generic functions, even though decisions made at senior levels have the most dramatic effect on the organization (Rakich, Longest, & Darr, 2000). Managers can be described by the functions they perform, the skills they use, the roles they play, and the competencies they must have to succeed. This emphasizes the process of managing.

Management Functions and Decision Making

The five management functions of planning, organizing, controlling, directing, and staffing are brought to life and connected by *decision making*, which is itself a subset of the essential process for managers that is known as *problem solv-*

ing. Little that managers at all levels in an organization do falls outside the purview of the five management functions. Management theorists and practitioners may chose one or two of the five functions as most important, but this is not borne out normatively. When one considers the full range of what managers do (or should do) as they perform their work, concentrating on a few to the exclusion or diminution of the others will invariably cause problems for the organization.

Decision making is an inherent activity of managers, and they make decisions within and among the five management functions. Decision making is part of the process of problem solving, which also includes problem analysis. Performance of the management functions and the decision making of problem solving should be evaluated using explicit and measurable criteria. In addition to engaging in the five management functions, managers must utilize specific skills, play various roles, and evidence a number of competencies.

Managing and Leading

Some theorists and academicians distinguish managers and leaders, based on the view that managing is more caretaking and maintaining status quo (transactional) whereas leading is more visionary and dynamic (transformational). That distinction may be more important pedagogically than in practical application, however, especially at the organization's operating level. Senior managers must ensure effective current organizational activities *and* that an organization's future is envisioned. Using this vision, the organization can be transformed as needed.

As they work to achieve organizational objectives, managers use technical, conceptual, and interpersonal skills. These skills are applied in various proportions, depending on the manager's task and level in the organizational hierarchy. Usually, senior managers make greater use of conceptual skills, whereas middle- and entry-level managers use a more even mix of the three.

The research of Henry Mintzberg found that managers have different roles, the general categories of which include interpersonal, informational, and decisional. Each may be segmented. For example, the interpersonal role includes figurehead and influencer, informational includes monitor and spokesperson, and the decisional role includes entrepreneur and negotiator. Successful managers integrate these various roles and are likely to engage in them without making a clear distinction.

Another way to understand managers' work is to identify their competencies, some of which are found in the categorizations discussed earlier. Conceptual, technical managerial/clinical, interpersonal/collaborative, political, commercial, and governance competencies are used in different proportions by managers at various levels of the organization.

Management Skills and Roles

Figure 2-1 suggests the relationships of technical, conceptual, and human relations skills and shows their typical weighting at various levels. Specific situations require greater or lesser use of the skills at all levels of the organization.

Skills

- *Technical skills* are the abilities of managers to use the methods, processes, and techniques of managing (such as preparing a budget or a pro forma, planning a new process, or reorganizing a workgroup). Technical skills tend to decrease in importance as managers become more senior.
- *Conceptual skills* are the mental ability to see how various factors in a given situation fit together and interact. Seeing second- and third-order consequences of decisions and nondecisions is especially important. The need to use conceptual skills increases significantly as managers become more senior.
- *Human/interpersonal skills* include cooperating with others, understanding them, and motivating and leading them in the workplace. Human relations skills tend to become less important as managers become more senior.

Roles Managers engage in a wide variety of roles as they do their work.

- The *interpersonal* roles of figurehead, leader, and liaison derive from the formal authority of the manager.
- The *informational* roles include monitor, disseminator, and spokesperson. The informational roles have special significance in organizations in the health field, which are more complex and require effective communication. Access to information is a measure of power. Less secure and capable managers tend to hoard information or provide it only reluctantly, thus reinforcing their importance.
- As noted, decision making is integral to the management functions. There are various types of *decisional* roles, including entrepreneur, resource allocator, and negotiator. In this group, negotiation may be the most important and is an almost daily activity of managers.
- The *designer* role is similar to that of the management function of organizing. Managers at different levels will design various components of the organization.
- The *strategist* role is not unlike the manager's planning function. It suggests a specific focus on how to adapt their organizational domains to external challenges and opportunities.

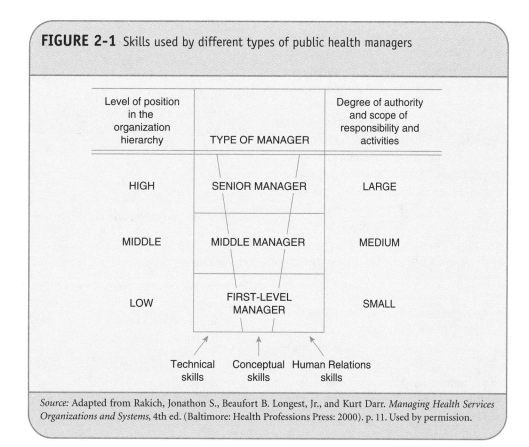

FIGURE 2-1 Skills used by different types of public health managers

Source: Adapted from Rakich, Jonathon S., Beaufort B. Longest, Jr., and Kurt Darr. *Managing Health Services Organizations and Systems*, 4th ed. (Baltimore: Health Professions Press: 2000). p. 11. Used by permission.

- The *leader* role is affected by how well the roles of designer and strategist are performed. The leader role is more difficult because of the dynamism of the health services field, the multiple constituencies of its organizations, and the potential need for extensive sharing of the leader role.

Competencies In addition to the classical management functions and managerial roles, managers must develop a number of competencies.

- *Conceptual competence* is like that of the conceptual role. Middle and entry-level managers use conceptual competence to understand how their work fits into the larger organization, as well as the interrelationships in their areas of responsibility. As suggested earlier, senior managers use their ability to conceptualize to predict consequences of decisions and nondecisions.
- *Technical managerial/clinical competency* enables managers to perform the work of management, as well as understand and more effectively direct the work in the unit(s) for which they are responsible. Managers without a clinical or technical background must make a determined and persistent effort to understand the basics of specialized activities in their areas of responsibility, as well as in the organization generally.
- *Interpersonal/collaborative competency* requires that managers have good interpersonal and collaborative skills so as to effectively lead or direct others. These skills enable the manager to instill a common vision, stimulate a determination to pursue the vision, and meet the objectives that are part of the vision.
- *Political competency* means senior-level managers must understand and be able to work with the political processes of local, state, and even federal government. Effective application of this competency is key to meeting the health needs of the community. The position and technical knowledge held by senior managers enables them to influence the legislative and rule-making (regulatory) processes.
- *Commercial competency* and economic success require that organizations create economic exchanges that offer value to those involved. Managers must establish and maintain an environment that facilitates these economic exchanges. This necessitates a businesslike orientation for basic operation, but with a humanitarian and Samaritan overlay. Many not-for-profit and government organizations fall prey to an overemphasis on doing good and neglect the need to manage in a businesslike fashion.

- *Governance competence* means working with the governing body[1] to establish a vision, assemble resources, lead the organization, and ensure accountability to stakeholders. These efforts require that senior managers interact effectively with members of the governing body. The governing body determines the right thing (direction) for the organization; management determines the right way to achieve it. Many chief executive officers (CEOs) are voting members of their governing bodies, or, if not, they attend governing body meetings and sit on its committees. Regardless, they interact with governing body members in various settings and in a variety of ways.

Leadership Behavior

Managers as leaders influence followers to achieve objectives because they have authority or power. Various sources of power have been identified: legitimate (formal), reward, coercive, expert, and referent. These sources of power are more likely to be complementary than mutually exclusive. Effective leaders understand the risks and benefits of using each type of power and try to use them appropriately. Some researchers have sought to explain leader success by identifying *leader traits* such as assertive, cooperative, decisive, and dependable, and *leader skills* such as intelligent, conceptually skilled, creative, and persuasive. Other researchers focused on leader styles, such as Rensis Likert (1903–1981), whose continuum of leadership effectiveness spans autocratic, benevolent, consultative, and participative/democratic.

An approach asserting that traits, behaviors, and styles are inadequate to explain the success of leaders is called *situational* or *contingency theory*. Its hypothesis is that certain actions or responses (behavior/styles) in some situations lead to success, while their use in other situations causes failure. Incorporating situational factors or contingencies into the analyses of leader styles made them more sophisticated and enhanced their usability. Many of the efforts to analyze leaders and the reasons for their success overlap, but they all contribute to understanding managers qua leaders (Rakich et al., 2000, ch 15).

Management Functions

Figure 2-2 shows the management functions and their intimate connection with decision making. None is necessarily more important than another. They are complementary and tend to have a sequence of use and connection. The dynamic

---

[1] *Governing body* is a generic term used to describe the body to whom the public health manager is accountable, whether it is a city council, county council, commissioners elected by a special tax district, commissioners appointed through an interstate compact, or the like.

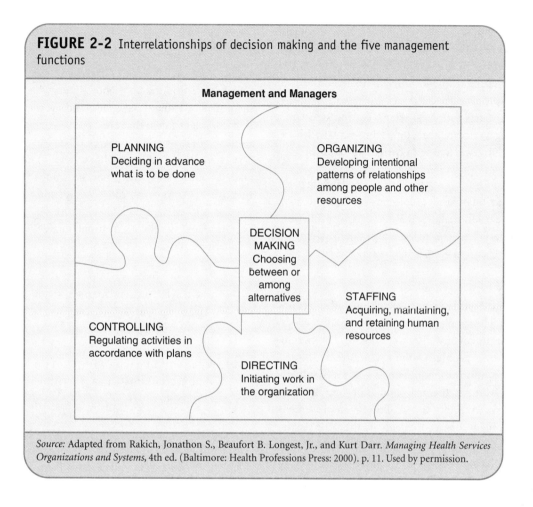

FIGURE 2-2 Interrelationships of decision making and the five management functions

Management and Managers

PLANNING
Deciding in advance
what is to be done

ORGANIZING
Developing intentional
patterns of relationships
among people and other
resources

DECISION
MAKING
Choosing
between or
among
alternatives

STAFFING
Acquiring, maintaining,
and retaining human
resources

CONTROLLING
Regulating activities in
accordance with plans

DIRECTING
Initiating work in
the organization

Source: Adapted from Rakich, Jonathon S., Beaufort B. Longest, Jr., and Kurt Darr. *Managing Health Services Organizations and Systems*, 4th ed. (Baltimore: Health Professions Press: 2000). p. 11. Used by permission.

that connects them is complex, and it may not be clear at any one time which function the manager is applying.

- *Planning.* Planning is usually identified as the first step of managing. It may occur *de novo* such as the planning for a new program, service, or facility. In addition, planning may be necessary after the outcomes of previous initiatives are found inadequate. Managers at all levels plan— although the focus, context, and terms are different.
- *Organizing.* Planning establishes objectives. Organizing develops intentional patterns of relationships among staff and other resources in the health services organization (HSO) to achieve these objectives. The result is an organizational design. There is a hierarchy in this design, beginning with individual positions and moving through work groups into larger units and, perhaps, eventually into an entire organization. The design of this hierarchy includes assigning authority and responsibility. Departmentation results from organizational design. Processes and integration are key to successful design.

- *Staffing.* Managers may give little thought to human resources until there is a problem with staffing, which includes acquiring, maintaining, and retaining human capital in the organization. Staffing is both technical (such as planning, job analysis, performance evaluation, and compensation and benefits) and social (such as training, promotion, and counseling). Given that the majority of costs in a typical organization are staff pay and benefits, it is difficult to overstate the importance of the staffing function.
- *Directing.* Directing occurs when managers initiate action. Effectively directing depends on being able to lead, motivate, and communicate with the staff for whom one is accountable. The various demands of effectively leading others necessitates a variety of leadership styles, some of which will be discussed later. The ability to motivate others is linked to having a shared vision.
- *Controlling.* The word suggests its function. At root, managers control by comparing actual with desired output and making adjustments. Controlling is directly

linked to planning, because the latter has set out the objectives that the organization (or its units) is expected to achieve, and controlling determines if this has occurred. Control monitors input and output, but it also monitors processes, or how work is done. Controlling has four basic steps: setting standards, measuring performance, comparing actual with expected results, and acting to correct deviations.

It is clear from Figure 2-2 and a basic understanding of the management functions that decision making is key to all of them. Without decision making, the management functions could not be undertaken. The process of problem solving inherent in most decision making is discussed next.

Problem Solving[2]

Middle- and senior-level managers spend most of their time solving problems. The results of problem solving affect allocation and use of resources as well as work results. The circumstances surrounding problem solving are often complex, unstructured, and nonroutine, thus making it difficult and time consuming. At times, the problem lies beyond the manager's direct control. Except for the condition of improvement, the process of problem solving is essentially the same regardless of problem type, scope, time involved, intensity of analysis, or the conditions that initiate it. Problem solving includes:

1. Problem identification, or recognizing the presence of a problem (including gathering and evaluating information) and stating the problem.
2. Making assumptions, which uses logic to extend what is known.
3. Developing tentative alternative solutions and selecting those to be considered in depth.
4. Evaluating alternative solutions by applying decision criteria.
5. Selecting the alternative that best fits the criteria.
6. Implementing the solution.
7. Evaluating the results of implementing the solution.

These steps are shown in **Figure 2-3**. The numbers in that figure correspond to those in the following discussion.

Problem Analysis [1] Problem analysis is divided into [1a] problem recognition and definition, and [1b] developing a problem statement. The product of problem analysis is the

problem statement. It is the problem statement about which assumptions are made in step [2].

Problem Recognition and Definition [1a] Problem solving under the condition of deviation occurs when actual results are inconsistent with desired results and the manager determines that this is a problem that must be solved. Examples of desired results are (1) organizationwide objectives such as quality of services provided or financial solvency; (2) program objectives such as increasing customer satisfaction, reducing staff turnover, or improving case finding; and (3) improving the performance of an individual employee.

Applying the theory of problem recognition is not easy. Problem recognition

> rarely occurs as a completely discrete event. In practice the process occurs through various time intervals (from seconds to years), amidst a variety of ongoing activities and in different ways depending on both situational and individual factors. At times, the process of problem recognition is automatic; at other times, it involves conscious effort. Often, it is a highly objective phenomenon resulting in problem descriptions that most anyone would agree on. At other times it is definitely a subjective process, where the nature of a problem description varies from individual to individual (Cowan, 1986, p. 764).

Problem recognition occurs in three stages. The first is *gestation/latency*, in which some cue or triggering event indicates a potential problem. The second is *categorization*, in which managers become aware that something is wrong but cannot clearly describe it. *Diagnosis* is third, which involves efforts to obtain the information that will provide greater certainty in problem definition (Cowan, 1986, p. 766). Often, symptoms clutter and confuse and make it difficult to recognize a problem and define its parameters. More experienced and expert managers are likely to be better problem solvers because they have superior problem recognition and definition skills. Asking the right questions, recognizing limits, and being sensitive to identifying and interpreting cues are skills gained only with experience.

Problem recognition and definition includes gathering, systematically evaluating, and judging the importance of information from sources such as routine reports and data, interviews and observation, information from workgroups, and customer feedback (Andriole, 1983). In this process, it is difficult to overestimate the importance of facts—information derived from consistently applied operational definitions. An

[2]Adapted from Chapter 7 of Jonathon S. Rakich, Beaufort B. Longest Jr., and Kurt Darr, *Managing Health Services Organizations and Systems*, 4th ed. (Baltimore: Health Professions Press, 2000).

FIGURE 2-3 Problem-solving process model

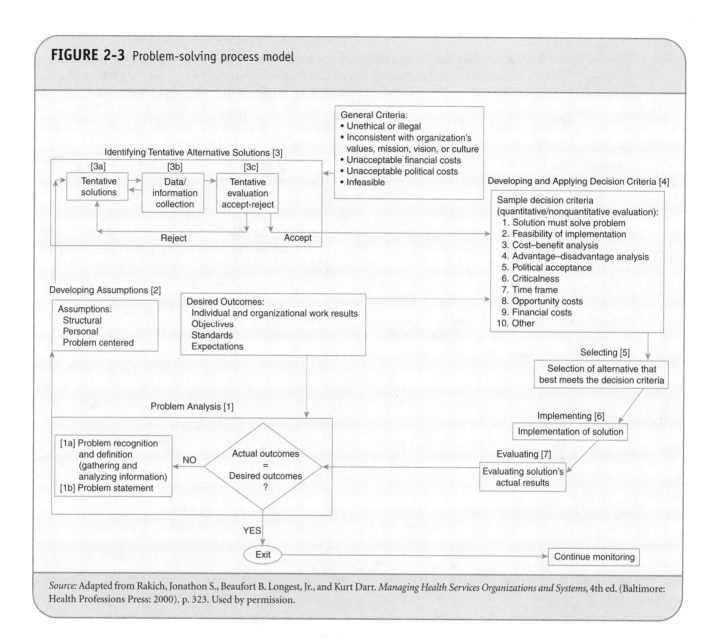

Source: Adapted from Rakich, Jonathon S., Beaufort B. Longest, Jr., and Kurt Darr. *Managing Health Services Organizations and Systems*, 4th ed. (Baltimore: Health Professions Press: 2000). p. 323. Used by permission.

essential and difficult job for the problem solver is to distinguish facts from other types of information—a learned ability honed by experience that improves problem solving.

In unstructured or complex situations, circumstantial evidence and deductive reasoning are helpful. Exclusionary thinking may be used to "rule out" problems. Once conclusions are reached, the problem is classified by type, nature, and scope. This recognition-definition stage is formative because subsequent actions, especially developing alternatives, are derived from it (Nutt, 1991). Ending the problem definition stage too soon will likely result in a low-quality solution or in solving the wrong problem (Chow, Haddad, & Wong-Boren, 1981).

Problem Statement [1b] The problem statement puts what is learned during the definition stage into a brief description of the problem to be solved. Almost always, one sentence is sufficient. Good problem statements have four parts: (1) an invitational stem, (2) an ownership component, (3) an action component, and (4) a goal component (Evan, 1991). The following sample problem statement contains the four parts: "In what ways can we improve system response time to reduce how long customers must wait for an answer to an inquiry about school vaccination requirements?"

In what ways can (stem)
we (owner of problem)

improve (action)

response time to reduce how long customers must wait for an answer to an inquiry about school vaccination requirements? (goal) (Couger, 1995, p. 184)

The invitational stem "In what ways can we ...?" encourages a divergent response, rather than the more narrow "How ...?" *Divergent* means thinking in different directions or searching for a variety of answers to a question that may have many right answers (Couger, 1995, p. 113).

The problem statement should have other attributes as well. Ideally, the problem definition phase has identified the root cause, which is reflected in the problem statement. If the problem statement reflects only a symptom, rather than the root cause, the problem must be "solved" again and again. A clinical simile is the symptomatic relief that aspirin gives flu sufferers; they feel better, but the cause is uncured. Sometimes, the root cause of the problem cannot be determined, or, even if the root cause is known, resources may be insufficient to solve it. Occasionally, it is politically infeasible to solve the root cause. There may be many reasons addressing symptoms is the only realistic choice. Doing so, however, must be seen for what it is— a temporary, expedient solution.

The problem statement should be narrow enough so that solving it lies within the problem solver's authority, resource limits, and the like, but not so narrow that only the symptoms are "treated." For example, certain employees seem to be taking too many coffee breaks. A narrow problem statement focuses on those employees. A somewhat broader problem statement addresses coffee breaks or breaks in general. An even broader problem statement, but one that is not too broad, identifies the efficient use of time or the quantity and assignment of work as the focus for action. Focusing on the employees addresses only a symptom, not the root cause.

The breadth of the problem statement also determines the clarity of direction that is given the problem solver. Narrow problem statements identify clearly what problem needs solving but risk addressing only a symptom. Overly broad problem statements may leave the problem solver without clear direction—no understanding of the first step. Sometimes problems are amorphous or lack specificity, especially as to knowing where to start. Organizational malaise or morale problems are amorphous. Here, problem solvers must cast their nets widely and engage in several iterations of problem solving— from the very broad to the more narrow and specific—before the problem is identified. Iterative problem solving is also known as heuristic problem solving.

The psychological stimulus that is provided by an action orientation should not be underestimated. Problem statements

include positive goals but may also include limitations. The problem statement regarding coffee breaks described earlier could be: "In what ways can I (we) solve the problem of excessive coffee breaks by staff so as to maximize use of staff resources, but without damaging morale?" Here, a limitation to be considered in selecting a solution is avoiding damage to staff morale.

There is more than one correct way to state a problem, but doing it well requires thought and the patience to prepare more than one iteration. The importance of developing a problem statement lies in the discipline of reducing thoughts to writing and the advantages of a written document in communicating to others who are working to solve the same problem. As the great American educator, John Dewey (1933), stated, "A question well put is half answered." The admonition to "Just stand there, don't just do something" until a suitable problem statement has been developed has more application than might be generally thought.

Facts and Reasoning A *fact* can be defined as an actuality, certainty, reality, or truth. Facts are highly prized and provide the firmest grounding for problem solving and decision making. Some facts are objectively verifiable. Many "facts" are subject to dispute, however, unless they result from an operational definition. Deming (2000) stressed the critical importance of operational definitions. Objectively verifiable facts or facts that are based on the same operational definition take precedence over all other types of information.

Once facts have been identified, two other issues arise. One is the weight to be given to them. Obviously, some facts are more important than others, and people who share problem-solving responsibilities must understand how facts are weighted. A second issue is that facts are subject to judgment and interpretation. For example, a tape measure will gauge a room's dimensions. Whether the room is large enough for a certain activity or job is a matter of opinion. The fact that the room has seating does not answer the question of how comfortable the seating is. Decision makers must be able to separate fact from conclusion (judgment), interpretation, and opinion and not allow them to merge.

Rarely are facts sufficient to solve a problem, however. Obtaining facts is necessarily constrained by time and resources. Problem solvers can partly overcome this deficit through inductive and deductive reasoning. *Inductive reasoning* moves from the single event or fact to a conclusion or generalization based on that event or fact. Inductive reasoning allows one to conclude that the fact of a painted wall means that there was a painter. *Deductive reasoning* uses the facts of related or similar events to reach a conclusion. Deductive reasoning is employed in a criminal prosecution when circumstantial evidence is used to prove the defendant's guilt, despite lack of direct evidence such as fingerprints or the testimony of a witness. Circumstantial evidence is based on inferences (deductions) that are drawn from facts. A deduction from finding room after room with half-painted walls is that the work of the painter(s) is undone.

Often, problem solvers and decision makers have the need to consider what weight, if any, to give to information that is hearsay, rumor, or assertion. "Hearsay" refers to words attributed to a third party. With few exceptions, hearsay is inadmissible in court proceedings. Similarly, decision makers should identify hearsay and give it little or no weight. Rumors abound in all organizations; many of them come to the notice of decision makers. They, too, should be given little weight. Assertions may be based on fact, hearsay, or rumor. Assertions may also be called judgments or conclusions. Assertions may be stated forcefully and with a degree of authority that seems to give them credibility. They must be accepted with caution.

Hearsay and rumor may have elements of truth. This makes them important to the extent that they suggest potential problems that warrant further investigation. In themselves, hearsay and rumor are never the basis for action or decision making. Persons who make assertions should be asked how the assertions are supported by facts. In the absence of facts, assertions should be given little or no weight.

Developing Assumptions [2] The problem statement developed in the problem analysis [1] allows the next step, developing assumptions [2]. Assumptions never supersede facts. When facts are insufficient, however, problem solvers use inductive and deductive reasoning to make assumptions. Only in the most unusual circumstances should problem solvers make assumptions that are unsupported by facts or logic because doing so means that the assumptions were chosen capriciously, which is not a basis for good management. Assumptions extend what is known. For example, if every time an employee is disciplined there are rumors that staff members will unionize, deductive reasoning tells us that the same thing will likely happen next time. This, then, is a logically supportable assumption.

Assumptions have a significant effect on the choice and quality of the solution and, consequently, on the quality of problem solving. In general, assumptions are of three types: structural, personal, and problem centered (Brightman, 1980).

Structural assumptions relate to the context of the problem—they are boundary assumptions: the problem lies within (or outside) a manager's authority; additional resources are (or are not) available to solve the problem; other departments cause the problem; or the problem is caused by an un-

controllable external factor—high unemployment in the county means that fewer people have employer-based health insurance and they must rely on public clinics for routine care.

Personal assumptions are conclusions and biases that decision makers bring to the problem. Often, they are based on experience. Managers may have a high or low tolerance for the risk and uncertainty inherent in changes that invariably result from problem solving. A manager's previous experience of being blamed for any problems caused by changes after problem solving may cause an aversion to risk, and this may lead to making assumptions about the problem or alternatives that cause selection of low-risk solutions. Assumptions may be made about the likely reactions of superiors, subordinates, or stakeholders to potential solutions. In addition to risk taking and other types of experiences that cause bias in the decision maker, the personal assumptions of anchoring and escalating commitment can affect problem solving. Anchoring occurs when the individual "chooses a starting point (an 'anchor'), perhaps from past data, and then adjusts from the anchor based on new information" (Chow et al., 1991, p. 194). An inaccurate anchor causes flawed analysis. Using last year's budget as a starting point for a new budget is an example of anchoring. Despite the problems, "[d]ecision makers display a strong bias toward alternatives that perpetuate the status quo" (Hammond, Keeney, & Raiffa, 2006, p. 120). The personal bias of escalating commitment means that a manager is unwilling to admit earlier mistakes. Managers whose decisions have become a problem "tend to be locked into a previously chosen course of action" (Chow et al., 1991, p. 202). The tendency of decision makers to make decisions in a way that justifies past choices has also been described as the "sunk-cost trap," meaning that old investments of time and resources cannot be recovered, but further commitments are made because it is so difficult for managers to admit past mistakes (Hammond et al., 2006, p. 122).

Problem-centered assumptions cover a wide range, including perceived relative importance of the problem, degree of risk posed by the problem, and how urgently a solution is needed. Other problem-centered assumptions include economic and political costs and benefits, the degree to which subordinates or superiors will accept solutions, and the likelihood of success if a solution is implemented.

It is important to emphasize that the three types of assumptions affect the decision maker and the problem-solving process differently. Assumptions differ in at least two ways: qualitatively, and in the amount of control that decision makers have over them. For example, a structural assumption that no funds are available to solve a problem profoundly affects the solutions that can be considered, and there may be little or nothing the decision maker can do to remedy a lack of funds. A personal assumption in which the decision maker recognizes an aversion to risk can be overcome to some extent, even though the decision maker may remain less willing to accept certain solutions or continues to be reluctant to experience higher levels of discomfort. Problem-centered assumptions are likely to involve more judgment, which is more often based on the decision maker's experience, hunch, or intuition, than are structural assumptions.

In summary, making assumptions is necessary to almost all problem solving. Decision makers must use caution in formulating and accepting assumptions because, if this step is done poorly, assumptions can limit the scope of problem solving or even preclude identifying the best solution (Chow et al., 1991).

Identifying Tentative Alternative Solutions [3] Once the manager has recognized, defined, and analyzed the problem; established its cause(s) and parameters; prepared a problem statement [1]; and made assumptions [2], tentative alternative solutions are developed [3]. In Figure 2–3 this step includes identifying tentative alternative solutions [3a]; collecting data/information [3b], if necessary; and evaluating the merits of each tentative alternative [3c] for an initial accept/reject decision. The initial accept/reject decision uses general criteria such as whether the tentative solution is unethical or illegal; is inconsistent with organizational values, mission, vision or culture; has unacceptable financial or political costs; or is infeasible. If no tentative alternatives meet these general criteria, the step must be repeated. Unique, nontraditional, and creative tentative solutions are identified more readily if structural, personal, and problem-centered assumptions are not overly restrictive.

Identifying tentative solutions is very important because it consumes more resources than any other problem-solving activity and because, if creativity is to occur, it must occur here (Nutt, 1993). It is in the tentative alternative solution loop that creativity is important (Couger, 1995). Although the terms are often used synonymously, *creativity*—defined as imagination and ingenuity—should be distinguished from the narrower concept of *innovation*—defined as changing or transforming (Couger, 1995).

Several categories or tactics that can be used to identify ideas for solutions have been described (Nutt, 1993). Regrettably, most do not suggest creativity as a source. *Ready-made tactics* assume that organizations have a store of fully developed solutions—a situation in which solutions wait for problems. *Search tactics* identify solutions from available ideas. Proposals are elicited and compared to identify solutions that seem viable. A *design tactic* seeks a custom-made solution—an opportunity for creativity.

Several factors influence the time and resources that are devoted to the tentative alternative solution loop. Most important are the quality and precision of the initial problem definition and the restrictiveness of assumptions. Others include sophistication of the organization's information systems, availability of data, and the degree to which the problem is structured. Unstructured problems are more complex, involve many variables, and take longer to solve than problems that are straightforward, relatively obvious, or narrowly defined. Typically, unstructured problems require several iterations of problem solving.

The tentative alternative solution loop has two hazards. Some managers spend excessive time and resources seeking the optimal solution when another solution is acceptable. In addition, extensive attention to activities in the loop and reiteration may be an excuse for not taking action. "I need more information" may be an excuse to procrastinate and make no decision (Etzioni, 1989).

Developing and Applying Decision Criteria [4] The alternatives that met the general criteria applied in the tentative alternative solution loop [3] are now ready for formal assessment. To select the best of several alternatives, managers must develop decision criteria that allow alternative solutions to be evaluated and compared [4]. The decision criteria include those in the "Desired Outcomes" cell in the center of Figure 2–3: individual and organizational work results, objectives, standards, and expectations. At least three other decision criteria are usually applied: effectiveness of the alternative in solving the problem, feasibility of implementation, and acceptability of the alternative based on objective and subjective analyses (Pearce & Robinson, 1989).

Alternatives that are not effective in solving the problem should be rejected. Examples are alternatives that solve only part of a problem, address only symptoms, or are not permanent. Exceptions may be necessary, however. For example, if the need for action is critical, it may be appropriate to select and implement a less-than-optimal solution because the consequences of doing nothing or waiting for a better solution are worse.

The feasibility of implementing an alternative is the second common decision criterion. Infeasible alternatives will be rejected in the tentative alternative solution loop. Those that survive may be implemented to varying degrees in terms of effort; structural boundaries and constraints; dependence on other people, departments, or both; and costs. Managers are less likely to select an alternative that depends on people and departments beyond their control. This is especially true if high political costs are associated with forcing implementation.

The third common criterion judges the effective use of resources, including quantitative (objective) cost-benefit analysis and assessment of nonquantitative (subjective) advantages and disadvantages. Lowest cost should not be a sole criterion—costs and benefits of alternatives must be considered, as should the opportunity costs of doing nothing. Objective evaluation means quantifying costs and benefits and should be attempted, despite the difficulty of estimating some data. Subjective evaluation means understanding advantages and disadvantages that may be impossible to quantify but cannot be ignored. Both types of assessment should be considered when evaluating and comparing alternatives. If an alternative is costly but the problem solver concludes that subjective considerations are more important, then a rational decision has been made. Here, it might be useful to list nonquantitative advantages and disadvantages, which adds the useful dimension of subjective judgment to the decision-making process.

Some decision criteria are likely to be more important than others in a given situation; several methods may be used to differentiate them. One method rank orders decision criteria using decision-maker judgments. Another method divides criteria into mandatory (must be met) and wanted. A solution that does not meet a *mandatory* criterion is discarded. *Wanted* criteria are weighted by degree of desirability. The resulting weighted scores determine which solution is selected (Kepner & Tregoe, 1981). A third method assumes that all decision criteria are equally important (which is unlikely) and judges how closely or well each alternative meets them and assigns a numerical value. The highest total determines which alternative is chosen. A decision matrix is an excellent tool for arraying and comparing decision criteria and solutions. **Table 2-1** shows a sample decision matrix.

The virtues of numerically weighting decision criteria include forcing decision makers to compare and evaluate them, thus providing a basis for discussion in group decision making. It is important that the numbers are understood to be

the results of judgments by decision makers, judgments that could be challenged by reasonable people. This basis in subjectivity means that the numbers are, at best, approximations. This must be borne in mind during analysis.

As noted earlier, this step is sometimes called decision analysis. Most often, decision makers have several alternative solutions that can be used; it is a matter of determining which one best (fully or partially) meets the decision criteria. There are, however, other variations of decision analysis. Sometimes, there is only one solution and a yes/no, accept/reject decision must be made. Here, the analysis compares the proposed solution to a reasonable (perhaps idealized) model of what could or should be done to determine whether the solution is acceptable. At other times, there are no alternatives and the decision maker must decide how to accomplish a desired result. Here, the first step is to clearly define the objectives. Then, a set of components that will most feasibly and effectively meet those objectives is selected from all of the available components (Kepner & Tregoe, 1981).

Selecting, Implementing, and Evaluating the Alternative Solution [5, 6, and 7] Almost always a manager selects an alternative (makes a decision) [5]. This does not end the problem-

TABLE 2-1 Decision Matrix for Evaluating Alternative Solutions

Decision Criteria	Alternative Solution 1	Alternative Solution 2	Alternative Solution 3
Must meet these requirements:			
1. Solution effectively solves the problem	3	5	5
2. Feasibility of implementation	5	3	5
3. Cost-benefit analysis	5	5	3
4. Advantage-disadvantage analysis	3	3	5
Wants to meet these requirements:			
5. Political acceptability	1	3	3
6. Criticalness	1	3	5
7. Time frame	1	3	5
8. Opportunity costs	5	1	3
9. Monetary costs	3	5	5
Total Score	27	31	39
Conclusion: Alternative solution 3 accepted.			

Key:
5 = Solution fully meets decision criterion.
3 = Solution partially meets decision criterion.
1 = Solution fails to meet decision criterion.

Source: Adapted from John D. Arnold, *The Complete Problem Solver: A Total System for Competitive Decision Making* (New York: John Wiley & Sons.,1992), p. 62.

solving process, however. Implementation [6] and evaluation [7] must be planned. Implementation [6] usually requires that resources are made available. The effects of the intervention (change) that has been implemented must be evaluated (monitored) [7] to determine that they are consistent with desired results [1]—the problem has been solved. Effective implementation and evaluation require that who will do what, how, and in what time frame are determined prospectively. It is desirable for evaluation to be integral (built in) to implementation. Data collection must be specific, especially as to where in the organization it will be done and with whom responsibility lies.

Evaluation is a commonly neglected part of problem solving—busy managers assume that the solution selected and implemented will be effective, and they turn to solving other problems. The solution, however, may solve the problem completely, partially, or not at all. Effectiveness of the solution can only be known if data are collected.

If the problem is not solved then the problem-solving process begins again, perhaps by fine-tuning the alternative implemented, reconsidering alternatives previously rejected, or developing new alternatives. Furthermore, solving one problem often causes others. For example, increasing the effectiveness of well-baby care may result in more case findings that require referrals to other providers, thus increasing costs of follow-up. This ripple effect necessarily leads to new rounds of problem solving.

Implications for the Public Health Manager

Problem solving is a major responsibility of managers at all levels. When done effectively, resource allocation and consumption are superior and results are more consistent with those desired. Managers' skills in problem solving, including decision making, are directly reflected in the quality of solutions and interventions.

Designing Formal Organizations

The organizing function, which encompasses the design (and redesign) of organizations, has its genesis in the planning function. Senior managers and, depending on the scope of decisions being made, the governing body are concerned with such broad aspects of organizing as authority and responsibility relationships, departmentation, and coordination and relationships of components whether within an organization or among the elements in a system of organizations. Lower-level (operational) managers are concerned with individual positions, aggregations of individual positions into workgroups, and clusters of workgroups. The work of classical management theorists such as Max Weber, Henri Fayol, and Chester Barnard established a theoretical basis for organizational design in the late 19th and early 20th centuries. Their concepts of division of

work, authority and responsibility relationships, departmentation, span of control, and coordination have been complemented by contemporary theorists. **Figure 2-4** shows levels of organization design.

Classical Concepts

The historical roots of organizational design theory—some of which date from the 19th century—continue to be important in contemporary management. Many design concepts can be traced to the hierarchy of the Roman Catholic Church and the organizational structures of European and American armies.

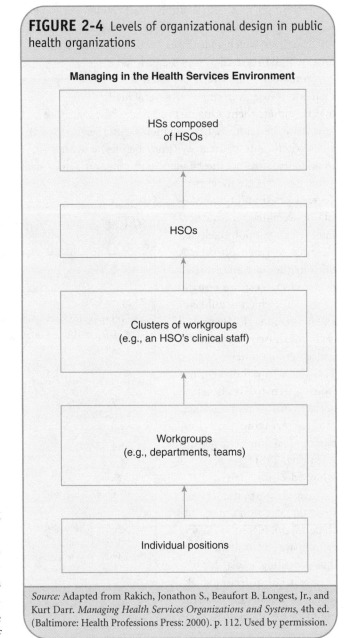

FIGURE 2-4 Levels of organizational design in public health organizations

Managing in the Health Services Environment

HSs composed of HSOs

HSOs

Clusters of workgroups (e.g., an HSO's clinical staff)

Workgroups (e.g., departments, teams)

Individual positions

Source: Adapted from Rakich, Jonathon S., Beaufort B. Longest, Jr., and Kurt Darr. *Managing Health Services Organizations and Systems,* 4th ed. (Baltimore: Health Professions Press: 2000). p. 112. Used by permission.

Weber and Bureaucracy

Max Weber (1864–1920) was the first to develop a theory about *bureaucracy*, which in its pure form was said to be the ideal and most rational form of organizing. The ideal bureaucracy included a clear division of labor, positions arranged in a hierarchy, formal rules and regulations to uniformly guide employees' actions, impersonal relationships between managers and employees, employment based on technical competence, and protection against arbitrary dismissal. Regrettably, bureaucracy has come to mean duplication, delay, waste, low morale, and low motivation. The word *pure* must be borne in mind when considering what Weber argued was desirable about bureaucracy.

Fayol and the 14 Principles of Management

Henri Fayol (1841–1925) identified 14 principles that he asserted were essential to management. These principles are often identified in management theory texts without naming Fayol as the originator. These principles seem intuitive and rational, yet they are often violated in organizational design and managing. Examples of these principles include division of work (specialization by tasks), authority (the ability to give orders), unity of command (employees should receive orders from only one person), scalar chain (a line of authority from top to bottom), and equity (managers should be kind and fair to their subordinates).

Machiavelli

Niccolo Machiavelli (1469–1527) likely did not consider himself a management theorist. His book, *The Prince*, written in the early 16th century described the problems of ruling and how rulers should deal with friends and enemies. He discussed the risks of being loved by subordinates, versus being feared by them, as well as the risks of being generous in payment and gifts. His insights are thought provoking and should be of interest to all serious students of management.

Division of Work

The concept of division of work can be traced to the economist Adam Smith, later reinforced by Fayol. It suggests the importance of *specializing* as a means of making workers more proficient and, thus, more efficient. Most organizations in public health have a high degree of specialization. Individual units might be very efficient, but it is the processes and interrelationships that are necessary for their work to be meaningful that become a problem. The value and concept of specialization are apparent in research findings showing that the quality of outcomes of service delivery declines as volumes go below certain minimums.

Authority and Responsibility Relationships

Authority is the power derived from someone's position in an organization. Implicit in this concept is that those with authority have an obligation to perform certain functions or achieve certain results and that that person is accountable to a higher level inside or outside the organization. Conversely, someone *responsible* for certain functions or certain results must have sufficient authority or power to achieve them. Managers fail if staff are held accountable for results of processes over which they have no control. Management must delegate authority proportionate to the responsibility (accountability) to which employees are held.

Departmentation

Departmentation results from the organization's need to specialize and the division of labor that specialization produces. The classical criteria groups workers into units and units into larger aggregations based on knowledge and skills, work processes and functions, time, output, client(s), and place (see Figure 2-4). The contemporary view uses bases such as service lines for departmentation. Service lines are developed because of the need to organize and deliver specific types of services. Decentralizing decision making, control, and goal setting further diminishes the perceived inflexibility of departmentation. Departmentation necessitates that management develop means of coordinating and integrating the work of departmented units.

Span of Control

The classical view of span of control is that there are inherent limits to the number of subordinates that can be effectively supervised. Smaller (narrower) spans of control result in taller organizations, that is, organizations with more levels. Larger (longer) spans of control result in flatter organizations. Some theorists set specific limits on how many subordinates could be effectively managed; others argued that the types of work to be done dictated the number of subordinates that could be managed. Regardless, it was agreed that effectively managing subordinates necessitated a limit on numbers. Organization of the Roman legions is instructive and quite precise as to the numbers and relationships, and undoubtedly contributed to their martial successes.

Coordination

The classical management theorist, Chester Barnard (1886–1961), noted that the quality of coordination is the crucial factor in survival of the organization. It is difficult to give coordination a more prominent place. The many specialized units—or silos—in organizations result in a great need for coordination. Committees, task forces, staff meetings, and voice and e-mail messaging facilitate coordination and highlight its importance. *Integration* is another word used to express the concept of coordination.

Contemporary Theorists

Peter F. Drucker

Peter F. Drucker (1909–2005) wrote extensively about managers, management, and organizations, and much of the conceptual framework for contemporary management theory derives from his work. For almost five decades after his first book, Drucker taught and wrote at Claremont College. Early training as a journalist and good knowledge of history and politics make his writing more akin to that of a novelist than a management theorist. Drucker's work as a consultant to large corporations allowed him to study organizations firsthand and develop observations about managers. His views on the traits of leaders are especially compelling. Drucker concluded that there may be charismatic leaders, but they are too few in number to make a difference. His experience persuaded him that successful leaders come in all shapes and sizes and have a wide range of personalities.

W. Edwards Deming

W. Edwards Deming (1900–1993) began his professional life as a statistician. He helped develop the theory of statistical quality control during the 1930s, a concept that was successfully applied to war production during World War II. In the late 1940s he taught Japanese industrial leaders how to use statistical quality control principles and systems thinking to produce high-quality consumer goods. Japan's success in this regard is obvious. Deming only received recognition for his work in the United States in the early 1980s, when he was featured in a public broadcasting special. Deming's 14 points for management focus on how organizations achieve quality. In his concept, managers have the responsibility to establish an environment with quality as the watchword and to improve processes so that quality can be achieved. Workers are inhibited in their efforts to produce high-quality goods and services by the processes that are developed, implemented, and controlled by management. Only management can foster improvement in services. Deming was an advocate of continuous quality improvement, a management philosophy that seeks to improve all processes in an organization. To Deming, quality improvement was not a program to be undertaken by a quality office. It is a philosophy that is customer driven and has the goal of meeting and exceeding customers' expectations.

Integrated Perspective

There is no one correct way to design an organization. More important is that the design or configuration selected furthers the goals of the organization. In this regard, it is useful to apply Drucker's criteria: clarity, as opposed to simplicity; economy of effort to maintain control; direction of vision toward the product, not the process; all individuals understanding their tasks and those of the organization; focused decision making; stability, not rigidity; and perpetuation and self-renewal.

MANAGEMENT PRACTICES

The formal organizational structure that managers design and implement provides important information about the planned interrelationships among its several elements. Within the formal structure, however, is the informal "organization," which consists of the numerous interpersonal relationships that develop outside the formal relationships established in the formal organization and that reflect the wishes and preferences of the people who work in the organization. The informal organization is characterized by dynamic behavior and activity patterns that occur within the formal organizational structure of people working together. These interactions and relationships arise spontaneously, but they are usually stable over time.

Informal groups give their members relief from monotony and boredom, offer interaction with persons having similar values, and allow achievement of a level of status that may be absent in formal relationships. Leaders emerge within informal groups. As is true with leaders of formal groups, leaders of informal group initiate action, resolve differences of opinion and conflicts, and communicate values to nonmembers.

Informal groups are most helpful to the formal organization when they blend with it. Other positive aspects include providing a level of flexibility while still meeting organization goals, providing social values and stability to the organization, allowing more general supervision, and facilitating communication. Effective managers understand and use informal groups to benefit the organization. Combined, the formal and informal organizations are the actual organization. Managers ignore informal groups and informal leaders at their peril.

Strategic and Operational Planning

Strategic planning addresses the longer-term direction and goals selected by the organization through its governance and management in order to accomplish its goals. Strategic planning may also be called strategic management, which suggests the broader, more dynamic concept of fully integrated management and planning. An extension of strategic planning that seeks to affect the external environment is strategic issues management (SIM). SIM is a systematic process that proactively seeks to influence the external environment to make it more favorable to the organization rather than reacting to events after they occur.

Operational planning focuses on the direction and activities of individual units and departments of the organization. The operational plan must be coordinated with and is subordinate to the strategic plan. **Figure 2-5** shows the general characteristics of strategic and operational planning.

Contingency Planning in Public Health

In their work, public health managers face many unknowns. *Contingency planning* seeks to predict the events that will affect the organization's ability to meet its mission; mitigates their potential negative implications; and, if possible, turns them into a public relations or political advantage. A well-known example of contingency planning in public health is planning for a natural disaster such as an epidemic of avian influenza or a manmade disaster such as a deliberate release of radioactive materials. These plans anticipate the demands of various scenarios, maximize effectiveness in response and minimize preventable morbidity and mortality. In addition, public health organizations must play a leading role in organizing the communitywide contingency planning for various types of disasters such as a severe earthquake, an outbreak of food poisoning that incapacitates large numbers, or a terrorist attack involving the release of poisonous chemicals. Communitywide contingency planning should also address interruption of utilities such as water, electricity, and natural gas. Failure to identify and plan for a variety of contingencies will prevent public

health organizations and providers such as hospitals from meeting their obligations to the public and will raise significant questions as to the quality of their management. At least in the military, it is said that the plan of battle has no value after the first engagement. The same is likely to be true for the contingency planning undertaken by the organizations concerned with the public's health. Besides obvious preparations such as periodic testing of communication links, emergency response and call-in drills, and knowing how to get emergency supplies of food and water, the public health organization's response must be flexible and developed with full recognition of the need for communitywide coordination and cooperation.

Managers as Negotiators

Successful managers are effective negotiators. The art of negotiating or bargaining applies to all internal or external transactions in which the parties decide what they will give and what they want to get. Negotiation is often characterized as win–win (cooperative) in which both parties benefit or win–lose (competitive) if one party prevails at the expense of the other. Deming argued that the result of win–lose negotiations is really lose–lose, because both parties lose.

Most negotiating in organizations is informal—for example, two managers agree to change how their departments coordinate activities. The result of these negotiations may be reflected in a memorandum, thus adding a level of formality. The most common type of formal negotiating occurs when contracts are negotiated and signed between or among parties who seek mutual benefit from the legal relationship that results. These contracts may be for the purchase of goods or services that are used as input to achieve its objectives, or they may bind organizations horizontally or vertically in relationships that they hope will benefit the public.

Typically, there are two sources of conflict in negotiating. The first is how the resources are to be divided—the money, goods, or services that are to be exchanged for what consideration. The second is resolving the psychological dynamics and satisfying the personal motivations of the negotiators in the organizations involved. The latter source of conflict is known as

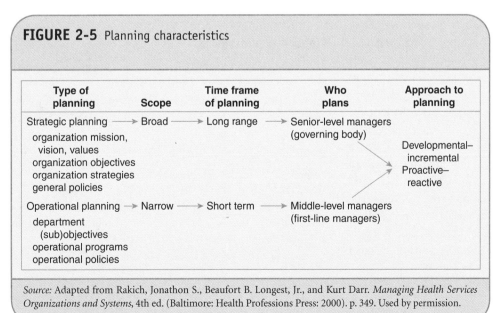

FIGURE 2-5 Planning characteristics

Type of planning	Scope	Time frame of planning	Who plans	Approach to planning
Strategic planning organization mission, vision, values organization objectives organization strategies general policies	Broad	Long range	Senior-level managers (governing body)	Developmental– incremental Proactive– reactive
Operational planning department (sub)objectives operational programs operational policies	Narrow	Short term	Middle-level managers (first-line managers)	

Source: Adapted from Rakich, Jonathon S., Beaufort B. Longest, Jr., and Kurt Darr. *Managing Health Services Organizations and Systems*, 4th ed. (Baltimore: Health Professions Press: 2000). p. 349. Used by permission.

the intangibles of negotiation and can include variables such as the ego involvement of appearing to win or lose, competing effectively, or cooperating fairly. The intangibles of negotiating are often the most difficult to understand and resolve (Rakich et al.).

Nonjudicial Means of Resolving Disputes

When disputes arise, legal action should be the last resort. There are far more efficient and lower-cost ways to settle disputes, whether they involve contracts, negligence (torts), employment, or interorganizational relationships. The methods used to settle disputes other than by recourse to the legal system are known as alternative dispute resolution (ADR). As described earlier, negotiation is not part of the ADR lexicon; it is, however, the first step managers should take to settle a dispute.

ADR has been widely used for decades to resolve commercial disputes; it is becoming more common to resolve disputes everywhere. ADR is private, inexpensive, and efficient—attributes that are especially important to organizations in the public and private sectors. ADR includes binding and nonbinding arbitration (which may be voluntary or involuntary), mediation, minitrials, neutral fact finding, and variations of these mechanisms. Each mechanism or variation has qualities that make it best for use in resolving a certain type of dispute. For example, mediation is especially useful when the parties want to have a continuing relationship. Binding arbitration may be contractually required by some state and local governments as a means of resolving disputes. There are for-profit and not-for-profit private organizations that provide panels of arbitrators, mediators, and other experts in ADR.

Both mediation and arbitration involve the use of a neutral third party. Mediators and arbitrators have very different roles and training, however. *Mediators* are neutrals who work with the parties to achieve a resolution of the dispute that is acceptable to them. Mediators have no authority to impose a settlement but use various techniques and persuasion to move the parties to a point where the dispute can be settled. The result is a contract between the parties that sets out the terms of the mediated settlement. Failing successful mediation, arbitration may be used as the next step in ADR.

Arbitrators are neutrals who are appointed pursuant to a contract signed by the parties to a dispute. The contract states that the parties will abide by the decision of the arbitrator. The arbitrator has authority to conduct a quasi-legal proceeding, gather evidence, and render a decision. The decision is legally enforceable by the parties because of the contract they signed agreeing to arbitration.

Measuring Managerial Performance

A balanced scorecard should be used to measure performance of the entire management team. Quantifiable outcomes should be emphasized, but not to the exclusion of a focus on meeting or exceeding customer expectations. This focus on customers will be a somewhat more difficult transition in government agencies and units that traditionally have a less-than-enviable record in this regard. In addition to a customer focus, managerial vision in terms of power, timing, and style is important.

Power

Public health managers are expected to use politics and power to achieve organizational goals. These managers build coalitions, make deals, and compromise collective goals to achieve as much as possible. These activities require managers to be highly political and engage in the pragmatic use of power. Here, it is important to understand politics as the art of the possible.

Timing

Change without crisis is a hallmark of good management, and effective managers identify issues far enough in advance to avoid a crisis. Understanding the demands and interests of the marketplace is essential in a consumer-driven public health system, which should be its goal.

Style

Management style is key to organizational success. Effective managers are predictable, frank, responsive and persuasive; can resolve conflicts; and encourage participation in decision making.

Importance of Values

It is difficult to overstate the importance of values. They will be considered in greater depth in Chapter 7. Successful managers have a clearly identified personal ethic, which they willingly share through word and deed. Organizations should recruit and retain staff at all levels based on shared values. Applicants must be screened in ways that emphasize what the organization stands for and the values context of its service delivery. These principles are even more important in selecting senior management who are expected to live and model a personal ethic that is consistent and that reinforces the organization's values.

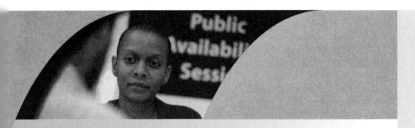

Discussion Questions

1. How do the organization's philosophy and its culture affect organizational performance? What is the role of managers in terms of the organization's philosophy and its culture?

2. Identify some of the differences and similarities in organization and management between public health organizations that are controlled by government and health services organizations in the private sector. Pay special attention to governance and organizational structure.

3. What is the relationship among the five management functions? Are some more important than others? If so, identify how and when.

4. How do managers develop the skills, roles, and competencies needed to effectively perform their work? Which of them cannot be learned?

5. Why is problem solving a generic skill? Provide some examples of problem solving from your professional or personal experience.

6. What considerations determine the design of an organization? Identify developments that necessitate changes in organizational design.

7. What is the role of negotiation in the work of managers? Identify examples of how alternative dispute resolution can assist a public health organization in achieving its mission.

REFERENCES

Andriole SJ. *Handbook of Problem Solving: An Analytical Methodology.* New York: Petrocelli Books; 1983:25.

A useful discussion of problem-solving constraints, including assumptions, is found in Brightman, HJ. *Problem Solving: A Logical and Creative Approach.* Atlanta: Business Publication Division, College of Business Administration, Georgia State University, 1980, chap. 3.

For a discussion on problem definition, see Chow CW, Haddad KM, Wong-Boren A. Improving Subjective Decision Making in Health Care Administration. *Hospital and Health Services Administration.* 1991;36(Summer):192–202.

Couger DJ. *Creative Problem Solving and Opportunity Finding.* Danvers, MA: Boyd & Fraser; 1995:113–184. An excellent discussion of techniques for generating solutions is found in Couger, *Creative Problem Solving,* chap. 8.

Cowan DA. Developing a Process Model of Problem Recognition. *Academy of Management Review.* 1986;11(Spring):764–766.

Dewey J. *How We Think: A Restatement of the Relation of Reflective Thinking to the Educative Process.* Boston: D.C. Heath; 1933:108. Quoted in Deming WE. *The New Economics for Industry, Government, Education.* 2nd ed. Cambridge, MA: MIT-CAES; 2000:104–105. "There is no true value of any characteristic, state, or condition that is defined in terms of measurement or observation. Change of procedure for measurement (change in operational definition) or observation produces a new number. . . . There is no true value for the number of people in a room. Whom do you count? Do we count someone that was here in this room, but is now outside on the telephone or drinking coffee? Do we count the people that work for the hotel? Do we count the people on the stage? The people managing the audio-visual equipment? If you change the rule for counting people, you come up with a new number. . . . There is no such thing as a fact concerning an empirical observation. Any two people may have different ideas about what is important to know about any event. Get the facts! Is there any meaning to this exhortation?"

Etzioni A. Humble Decision Making. *Harvard Business Review.* 1989;67(July-August):125.

Evans JR. *Creative Thinking in the Decision and Management Sciences.* Cincinnati, OH: South-Western; 1991:104.

Hammond JS, Keeney RL, Raiffa H. The Hidden Traps in Decision Making. *Harvard Business Review.* January 2006;84(1):120–122.

Kepner CH, Tregoe BB. *The New Rational Manager.* Princeton, NJ: Kepner-Tregoe; 1981:94–137.

Nutt PC. How Top Managers in Health Organizations Set Directions that Guide Decision Making. *Hospital and Health Services Administration.* 1991;36(Spring):59.

Nutt PC. The Identification of Solution Ideas During Organizational Decision Making. *Management Science.* 1993;39(September):1071–1072.

Pearce JA, III, Robinson RB, Jr. *Management.* New York: Random House; 1989:75. This text describes these criteria as Will the alternative be effective?, Can the alternative be implemented?, and What are the organization consequences?, respectively.

Rakich JS, Longest BB, Jr, Darr K. *Managing Health Services Organizations and Systems.* 4th ed. Baltimore: Health Professions Press; 2000:chapters 1, 15, 7, 5.

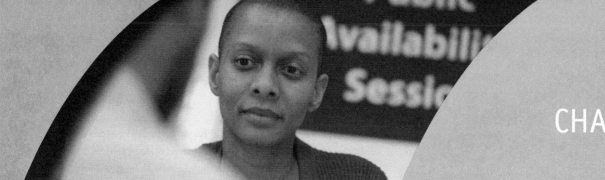

CHAPTER 3

Leading Public Health Organizations: Team Building, Reorganization, and Board Relationships

Leonard H. Friedman

INTRODUCTION

Managing in the public sector is frequently thought of as a team sport. In this case, leadership takes on the role of the coach. You have a roster of very talented employees who have to work together as part of a cohesive and highly effective team. In your role, you must have a clear understanding of how to build and support teams, drive teams to the highest levels of performance, and (in many cases) how to diagnose and deal with underperforming teams.

Every leader in every organization must be able to carefully examine the organization of people, services, and the flow of information. You have the opportunity to create an organizational design that is the optimal fit with the menu of services you provide and the needs of your stakeholders. Careful consideration of organization design will help you use resources more effectively, improve organizational communication, clarify roles and responsibilities, and better control your activities.

All public health organization leaders have to answer to a governing board. In some cases that board is a group of community volunteers, or it could be a group of elected officials. In either case, the relationship between the organization leadership and the governing board must be carefully thought out and managed. Your board is your boss and, as such, has the ultimate fiduciary duty for the organization. Managing the relationship between you and the board will be a critical component to your success.

LEARNING OBJECTIVES

After reading this chapter, the reader will be able to:

1. Describe the importance of groups and teams in public health organizations.
2. Outline the important aspects of the group process, including communication, leadership, stages of group development, and decision making.
3. Examine the factors associated with high-performing teams.
4. Understand the principles of organization design and the factors influencing the choice of organization design.
5. Distinguish among multiple types of organization design.
6. Describe the composition, key roles, and responsibilities of the governing board.
7. Discuss methods by which the leader can effectively manage his or her relationship with the governing board.

TEAMS

Take a moment and think about teams that you have either been on or have seen perform. These teams can be at work, at school, on the field of play, or as part of any number of other venues. What do you remember about those teams as being particularly outstanding? Some of those attributes might include:

- A focus on accomplishing a particular goal.
- The feeling that all the members of the team are operating as a single unit, where everyone knows what everyone else should do at that time.
- A willingness to set aside ego and personal ambition for the sake of the team.

- A high level of commitment and trust between and among team members.

While it might appear that it takes little or no effort to bring people together into highly functioning teams, nothing can be further from the truth. Growing and nurturing effective teams is a difficult and time-consuming task. To get the most from the teams in your organization, it is important that you attend to the following: understand and communicate the importance of teams in public health; have a clear view of the different types of teams, particularly in terms of the distinction between formal and informal teams; and enhance team effectiveness.

Importance of Teams in Public Health

Public health organizations are characterized by comparatively few staff members who must accomplish great things with very thin resources. Your staff is typically made up of a broad spectrum of workers, including clinical professionals, clerical staff, community volunteers, and even university interns. Funding is generally dependent on government appropriations, contract/grant income, or philanthropy. At the same time, the list of services that need to be provided by the organization (as in the case of a county health department) can be daunting. To get everything done with the human, financial, and technological resources available, it becomes necessary for people to work collaboratively with one another in team-based efforts. A number of examples of team activities come immediately to mind. Quality improvement efforts are structured around the ability of cross-functional teams to work with one another to manage every part of that process—from problem identification, to defining the work processes, to developing solutions, and finally to testing and implementing the best ideas. A disease outbreak requires that teams of specialists work effectively with one another in order to quickly identify the source of the problem and then to minimize its impact on the community. We intuitively know that teams are important in our work, but comparatively few of us have formal training on how to best structure and manage teams in order to achieve their maximum effectiveness.

Types of Groups and Teams

In the workplace, most of us have experience with formal groups in the form of committees, work teams, or other officially sanctioned team-based collections of people. We dedicate time to discuss these formal groups a bit later, but it is important to attend to the role of informal groups first. We should point out that we use the words *groups* and *teams* interchangeably.

Informal Groups

In virtually every organization, *informal groups* are created to fill some sort of social or personal interest or need. Think about the various types of informal groups that might be in your workplace: the people you ordinarily meet for lunch; the members of your carpool; those who make up your organization's softball or bowling team. What is it that brings these groups together and holds them together? There is typically no formal leader. There are no policies and procedures. Members who stay with the group conform to a whole series of unwritten norms governing their behavior. Generally speaking, informal groups tend to be fun and can be an important form of social support in sometimes overly formal and impersonal organizations.

In some cases, informal work groups can have a negative or potentially destructive outcome. An example of the downside of informal work groups is described by Amati Etzioni (1961, p. 114) in his classic description of informal groups in a factory setting:

> The workers constituted a cohesive group which had a well-developed normative system of its own. The norms specified, among other things, that a worker was not to work too hard, lest he become a "rate-buster"; nor was he to work too slowly, lest he become a "chiseler" who exploited the group (part of the wages were based on group performance). Under no circumstances was he to inform or "squeal." By mean of informal social control, the group was able to direct the pace of work, the amount of daily and weekly production, the amount of work stoppage and the allocation of work among members. In this instance, informal groups of employees were able to maintain social control as well as control over the pace of work through the imposition of informal, though well-enforced rules of behavior.

Have you seen this sort of thing in the workplace or ever been part of this type of informal work group? In your leadership role, you cannot ignore the presence of these informal groups. When they play a positive role, informal groups should be encouraged and nurtured. When these groups play a negative role, it could be an indication of employee and staff dissatisfaction. In either case, informal groups exist. Your job as a leader is to recognize their existence and understand that they can provide you with an important gauge of the health of your organization.

Formal Groups

For the purposes of this chapter, we will define *formal groups* as having the following characteristics: they have boundaries (generally written policies and procedures, rules and regulations, or formal bylaws), they have distinct member roles, there are specific tasks that are performed and measured, and they operate within a specific organizational context. These formal teams can be permanent, or they can be formed and dissolved after a short period of time.

While a ubiquitous part of organizational life, most people in an organization are ambivalent at best about teams. In light of all the literature about the value of teams in the workplace, why would this be the case? Perhaps you should ask your staff what they think about teams and their experience with workplace groups and teams. You will likely hear about time wasted, free-riders, dysfunctional groups, poor communication (including little or no listening to one another), boorish behavior, and out-of-control egos. Given this reality, your task as a public health leader is to understand how to craft and nurture teams that are effective, productive, and satisfying to their members.

Improving Team Effectiveness

A very comprehensive and easily understood model of team effectiveness was developed by Fried, Topping, and Edmondson (2006) and will serve as the framework upon which our discussion of team effectiveness rests. The model is pictured in **Figure 3-1**. In this model, team effectiveness is not a single point. Rather, there are multiple dimensions of ultimate effectiveness, including various performance measures such as greater efficiency (e.g., number of children vaccinated or measured improvement in access to health services for vulnerable populations). Performance is not the only possible measure of team effectiveness. The satisfaction of the team members is an important consideration and can significantly affect the willingness of the persons to work on this and other teams. If people have a positive experience and look forward to meeting with the other team members, there is a strong likelihood that the quality of work of the team will be enhanced. The final attribute of team effectiveness in the Fried model is the capacity for sustainability. Our concern should be how well the team can continue to work on the task at hand, particularly when considering the viability of a team that will stay together for an extended period of time.

In this model, effectiveness is a series of outcomes. All of these outcomes are affected by a whole set of process variables, which, in turn, are shaped by team characteristics, nature of the task, and environmental context in which the team is working. Process variables identified in the Fried model include (team) leadership, communication networks and interaction patterns, methods of group decision making, learning, and the need for every team to go through the stages of team development.

Leadership in teams is frequently seen as the ability to influence others toward the achievement of a particular goal or task. Depending on the composition of the group, one particular leadership style may be more effective than another. Regardless of the style of the leader, there should be a continual focus on the communication of clear goals, participation by all members of the team, provision of resources for the team to do its work, and a commitment to excellence. While there will frequently be a formal leader of the team (including department heads or

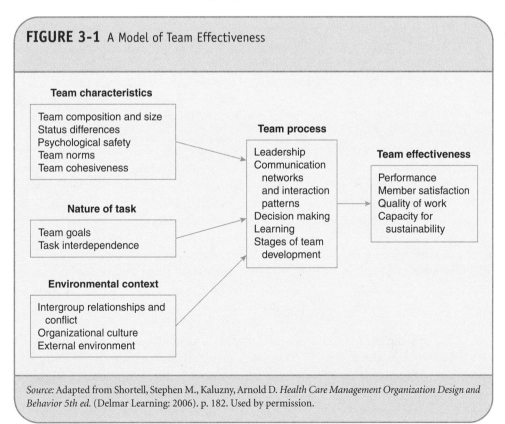

FIGURE 3-1 A Model of Team Effectiveness

Source: Adapted from Shortell, Stephen M., Kaluzny, Arnold D. *Health Care Management Organization Design and Behavior 5th ed.* (Delmar Learning: 2006). p. 182. Used by permission.

other management staff), just as often there will be informal leaders to whom members of the team look to for legitimacy and support.

Communication networks and interaction patterns are crucial elements of team processes. Without workable communication structures, important information may be lost or inaccurately communicated. How is communication in the team going to be facilitated? Is an intranet going to be used? Regular meeting updates? How about one-on-one conversations? One very good piece of advice came from the board chair of a health system that was in the process of merger talks with another hospital. The chair said that when you think you have communicated an important idea enough times, repeat it again and again. This idea of *redundant communication* is critical to reducing misunderstanding and making sure everyone is hearing the same thing.

Within the team, communication serves important process roles, specifically around maintenance and task behaviors (Bales, 1950). Maintenance behaviors in teams are activities that enhance interpersonal relationships and lead to open communication, support for team members, and conflict reduction. Task behaviors are those activities that relate specifically to completing the task at hand. Leaders of the team need to know and understand how communication can either facilitate or hinder maintenance and task behaviors.

All teams are involved at one time or another with *decision making*, and this is frequently a cause of significant intergroup conflict, particularly around how decisions are made. There is no one best way for a team to make decisions, and the choice of decision rules needs to be made explicit from the beginning. For some decisions, a simple majority might be enough. Some decisions might require two-thirds or more of the members to concur. Other decisions might be so important that there must be 100% concurrence. One of the important decision attributes that must be considered is the balance between data and speed. Every team needs to use data and information in order to come to a decision—yet a common trap is for certain teams to suffer "paralysis by analysis" or the unwillingness/inability to make a decision because there is always more data that can be collected and additional analysis that can be performed. How quickly does the decision need to be made? In a crisis situation, time is short but the team must be able to carefully consider its options.

Two other characteristics of team decision making should be addressed. The first is the "free-rider" effect (Albanese & Van Fleet, 1985). This is the person who obtains the benefits of group membership but does not accept a proportional share of the costs of membership. You have likely seen these people in

your own organizations. They are continually trying to promote their self-interest over that of the team or will not participate in any of the work associated with the team for a variety of different reasons. Yet, when all is said and done, this person will be happy to accept the credit given to the group for its efforts. As a manager, you need to address the behavior of the free-rider and uncover the incentives that he or she needs to fully participate in the team.

The other characteristic is a phenomenon known as "groupthink" (Janis, 1972), where a team prematurely moves to a poor decision. Groupthink occurs when the desire for harmony and consensus overrides the rational efforts of the members to think clearly about the situation. As a result, teams limit themselves to only one possible solution and fail to conduct a complete analysis of the problem. Leaders of teams need to work to avoid groupthink from even occurring. Members can be encouraged to speak up even if they have an opinion or assessment that is contrary to the rest of the group. All solutions should be critically evaluated. Strong and forceful individuals cannot be allowed to dominate a team and drive the decision process.

Group learning takes place when the collective skills, talents, and insights of the group come together in a way that allows the larger group to learn from its members and its environment in a way not available to individual members. Learning teams are more sensitive to subtle signals in their environments and can improve their understanding of the needs of internal and external stakeholders, improve their overall understanding of situations, and better deal with errors.

All teams go through a *development process* that generally (but not always) includes the following stages:

- *Forming*. This is the stage where the team members get to know one another and the purpose of the team. Members are generally polite with one another and interactions are somewhat forced and artificial.
- *Storming*. At this stage, the team is frequently in conflict as members try to influence norms, roles, and procedures.
- *Norming*. Teams at this stage are growing in cohesiveness and purpose as agreement on roles, expectations, and decision making take place.
- *Performing*. The team is most productive at this stage, where they move forward toward the accomplishment of agreed-upon goals and objectives.
- *Adjourning*. This is the stage at which temporary teams wrap up their work and disband. This stage is frequently met with sadness and regret (Tuckman, 1965).

Team Characteristics

The Fried model describes a number of characteristics that influence the team and ultimately affect the team's process and effectiveness. These include team composition, status differences, psychological safety, team norms, and team cohesiveness.

The *composition* of the team is an important consideration for all public health leaders. You need to ask yourself the following questions (Hackman, 1990):

- Is there adequate staff for the team, and is there adequate diversity (defined very broadly)?
- Do the team members have the expertise required to perform team tasks well?
- Are the members so similar that there is little for them to learn from one another? Conversely, are they so dissimilar that there is a risk of impaired communication and coordination with one another?
- Is the team made up of members who have worked together before? If not, will they need time to get to know one another?

Status differences can have an important effect on team members and their interaction with one another. We know that high-status members (e.g., physicians or senior managers) initiate communication much more often, are provided more opportunities to participate, and have more influence over the decision-making process (Owens, Mannic, & Neale, 1998). As a result, members from lower-status groups may be intimated or ignored by high-status members. The downside to this is that the group loses the insights and experience of a significant number of its members.

Psychological safety is a measure of the willingness of team members to take interpersonal risks and the beliefs they hold about the consequences of those risks, particularly when others disagree. Measures of psychological safety include the beliefs held by team members about how others will respond when they report a mistake, propose an idea that runs contrary to what the team has traditionally done, or even ask a question. In teams that have a high level of psychological safety, members are encouraged to experiment, ask other members for help, and talk about mistakes or errors without fear of retribution, shame, or guilt. Another benefit to teams that are psychologically safe is that the members of the team experience enhanced levels of learning and potentially higher levels of performance than teams where fear, anxiety, and suspicion are the rule.

Team norms are powerful influences on the behavior of individuals and groups. They are unwritten but fully understood attributes that govern and regulate behavior. Hackman (1976) suggests that norms have the following characteristics:

- They summarize and simplify team processes and regulate member behavior.
- They apply only to behavior and not to private thoughts and feelings. Private acceptance of norms is not necessary, only public compliance is required.
- They are generally developed only for behaviors considered important by the team.
- They usually develop gradually, but members can accelerate the process.
- All norms do not necessarily apply to all members. Some may apply only to newer members, while others can be applied on the basis of seniority, status, or economic class.

Team cohesiveness is a function of the extent to which team members are committed to the task of the group. You should note that the source of attraction is the task and not the individuals on the team. For persons in a public health environment, this can be a very important consideration and should be emphasized by management. Highly cohesive teams may have higher levels of performance, increased satisfaction by team members, and decreased turnover.

Nature of the Task

There are two important considerations about the nature of the task itself that the team has to confront: team goals and task interdependence.

Team goals and their accompanying tasks can be categorized according to goal clarity, complexity, and diversity (Fried et al., 2006). Take, for example, a task that is considered routine and predictable such as disease surveillance. In this case, the team members have clear and concrete goals, they have done this task before and know how the team should function, and the work of the team can almost appear to be routine. Conversely, imagine the response of your organization to a disaster. In this case, there is an extremely high level of uncertainty, bordering on chaos. While the macro goals of the team may be clear (depending on the precise team and the disaster being confronted), the micro goals may not be obvious at all. The team must almost "make it up as they go along," which can have terrible consequences. In this case, clear communication, the ability to rapidly adjust to changing environmental conditions, and ongoing coordination are vital.

Task interdependence is really nothing but a form of task diversity and speaks to the degree to which team members need to depend on one another in order to accomplish the task. The level of interdependence can grow from the individual, to the team, to the organization itself. In this case, higher levels of task interdependence translate to greater levels of uncertainty among the team members.

Environmental Context

Every team operates within an organizational environment that exerts pressure on the team and frequently affects the outcome of the team's process. In the model we describe, the *environmental context* is mediated by intergroup relationships and conflict, organizational culture, and the external environment itself.

In this case, *intergroup conflict* is defined as the conflict that arises when different teams are at odds with one another as opposed to the conflict that exists between or among members of a single team. In many instances, teams must coordinate their work with other teams. In any sort of organizational system, there will always be a level of turf protection, a desire to gather resources at the expense of other groups, and the tendency to blame others when things go wrong. In most organizations, teams and groups work to optimize conditions for themselves and do not understand the effect this suboptimization has on the larger system. Rather than look at what is best for the larger organization and the macro goals, teams that are in conflict with one another seek out win–lose strategies, where problem solving is replaced by the need to achieve victory for the group at all costs.

Given the importance of teams to be able to work effectively with one another, Fried and colleagues (2006) suggest a number of strategies, including:

- Intergroup training, including team-building exercises.
- Structuring the relationship between teams around mutually important goals.
- Carefully examining how teams interact to determine the sources of conflict.
- Reorganizing the teams into new groups that can work independently of one another.

Organizational culture is one of the most frequently voiced complaints about why teams fail to work as needed. Senior leadership says that they highly value team-based activities and then fail to provide the resources and support systems to allow teams to do their work. If senior leadership is truly going to create and sustain a culture that supports highly effective teams, continuous training must be part of the process. Imagine for a moment a sports team whose members are introduced to one another and then told to perform without any training, coaching, or other support. Why should we treat teams in public health settings differently or expect different results?

The final environmental context attribute is the *external environment* itself. Up until now, we have focused on the effects of the internal environment. While that internal environment is very important, the external environment cannot be ignored, and it can sometimes be even more important than the internal environment. For public health teams, perhaps the largest external environmental factor is the availability of funding to support the activities of the organization. Frequently, as a result of resource scarcity, members of public health organizations must depend on the goodwill of other organizations in order to get their work done. The ability to create and sustain relationships with outside partners is an important part of effective teams in resource-poor environments.

ORGANIZATION DESIGN

Several years ago, the movie *Field of Dreams* coined the oft-used phrase, "If you build it, they will come." What emerged from a cornfield in Iowa was a beautifully manicured and perfectly crafted baseball field, where the legends of the game appeared and rekindled old rivalries and old friendships. What if the character played by Kevin Costner decided instead to build a basketball court or perhaps a corn maze? Would the baseball players of old have emerged from the cornfields and played the game they all loved? Would building anything other than a baseball diamond have met the needs of those long-deceased players? The lesson from this example is that organization design is an intentional and purposeful process that seeks to position the building blocks of the organization in a way to help the organization achieve its mission, improve effectiveness, and best meet the needs of internal and external stakeholders. Organization design is a dynamic process and should be used as necessary. This portion of the chapter takes you through the fundamental principles of organization design, the factors that go into the choice of a particular organization design, and the various forms organizations can take.

Principles of Organization Design

There are a number of core principles of organization design that all persons in public health leadership roles should keep in mind:

- Organization design is never static. Once a design is decided upon and in place, it is only as good as the current environment dictates. Be prepared to change the design should original conditions change sufficiently.
- Allow a particular organization design to be in place so that you can evaluate whether or not it is most appropriate. Organization redesign is necessary, but, if done too frequently, it can lead to significant employee fatigue and loss of productivity.

- While we think of organization design as a rational process, things such as change in leadership, shifting organization goals, or changes in financial condition might dictate a particular design.
- Do not fall into the trap of thinking that there is one best organization design. Organization redesign is an ongoing process.
- The design process is a core part of management activities and must take into account authority, responsibility, accountability, resources (of all sorts), and rewards.

How do you know when it is time to think about redesigning your organization? The most important clue will be when you are experiencing significant performance problems, including employee and customer dissatisfaction, ongoing financial problems, excessive error rates, or other measurable items. These can be at the level of the work group, team, department, or entire organization. Another clue might be when an entirely new product or service is either introduced or is discontinued, particularly when that change results in significant additional funds coming into the organization. One other strong signal that redesign is called for is when there is a major shift in the organization's policies. This can come about by changes in government regulation or as a result of decisions made by the governing board. One final signal is a change in senior leadership in your organization. The fact is that sometimes a change in senior leadership gives an organization the opportunity to critically examine the ways that things have been done and ask what has or has not been working.

One of the classic models describing the fundamental principles of organization design was put forth by Henry Mintzberg (1983) (see **Figure 3-2**). Every organization is made up of five components of varying size and is surrounded by an ideology that has the potential to have an important impact on the people within the organization. The five parts to an organization are:

- *Strategic apex.* This is typically made up of the senior leadership, including the chief executive officer (or equivalent) and those few people immediately below the CEO on the organization chart.
- *Operating core.* These are the people who do the fundamental work of the organization. In a hospital, the operating core would be nurses and employed physicians. The operating core of a county health department would be the professional staff in each of the departments.
- *Middle line.* These are the people who connect the strategic apex with the operating core; it is typically populated by department managers.
- *Technostructure.* This is typically the technical staff whose work is required but is not central to the opera-

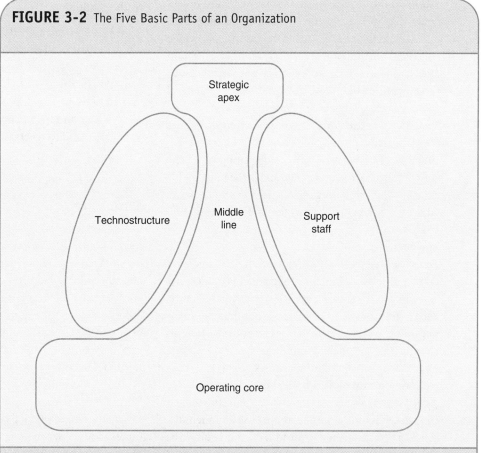

FIGURE 3-2 The Five Basic Parts of an Organization

Strategic apex

Technostructure

Middle line

Support staff

Operating core

Source: Mintzberg, H. (1983). *Structures in fives: Designing effective organizations.* Englewood Cliffs, NJ: Prentice-Hall. p. 11.

tion of the organization. In the example of the health department, the persons in the technostructure might be the staff of the information systems or legal department.

- *Support staff.* These people directly support the work of those in the operating core.

In addition to these five parts, all organizations have an ideology to one degree or another. For Mintzberg, ideologies represent the collection of beliefs, culture, norms, and values that inform the work of everyone in the organization. These mediators of ideology are discussed more thoroughly when we get to the factors influencing the choice of organization design.

These five parts could be arranged to result in five basic organizational forms:

- *Simple structure.* This structure is typical of start-up, entrepreneurial organizations. In this structure, there is nothing but a strategic apex and an operating core. Information flows easily from the managers to the workers. There is little or no hierarchy and there is little division of work with people doing multiple tasks.
- *Machine bureaucracy.* This is the organizational design in which standardization of work is absolutely required. This is generally seen in manufacturing, where consistency in output is at the heart of the organization and is governed by strict rules and regulations. Organizations like the U.S. Postal Service, General Motors, and McDonald's operate in this way.
- *Professional bureaucracy.* This organization also values standardization of work, but the focus is on the professional workers who occupy the operating core. The support structure is quite large and is the most highly developed of all the organizational forms. Hospitals, large physician clinics, county health departments, and large law firms are typically organized as professional bureaucracies.
- *Divisionalized form.* This organizational arrangement takes multiple machine or professional bureaucracies and controls them under a single ownership structure. Each of the units operates in a semi-autonomous manner but reports to the larger corporate parent. Examples of this include multihospital systems, state university systems, and companies like General Electric with multiple divisions who report to a single CEO.
- *Adhocracy.* These are temporary organizations that come together for a particular purpose and then dissolve. In this arrangement, the workers must quickly be able to adjust to one another and to the demands of the work. Examples of adhocracies are special project teams that pull out some of the best staff members

from across the organization to work on a project outside the auspices of the larger organization.

Now that we have examined the basic principles of organization design, we explore the factors that go into the choice of a particular organizational form.

Factors Influencing the Choice of Organizational Form

Before selecting the particular type of organization design that we would like to put into place, the astute public health leader must keep in mind a number of factors—all of which influence which design will be of greatest value to the organization. These factors include mission, environment, organization, culture, human resources, and politics (Fried et al., 2006).

Mission

The mission of any organization is a statement of its purpose or reason for being. It clearly tells stakeholders of all types exactly what the organization does. For example, a particularly well-written mission statement from the American Red Cross reads as follows:

> The American Red Cross, a humanitarian organization led by volunteers and guided by its Congressional Charter and the Fundamental Principles of the International Red Cross Movement, will provide relief to victims of disaster and help people prevent, prepare for, and respond to emergencies.

Any organization design chosen by the American Red Cross must be congruent with this mission.

Environment

One of the activities all smart and strategic organizations perform on a routine basis is an external environmental assessment. What is going on outside the organization that could affect overall organizational effectiveness? Public health leaders need to be cognizant of environmental changes in the areas of technology, legal and regulatory requirements, community demographics, worker supply and demand, and competitors, and make sure the choice of organization design provides the flexibility to adjust to these changes.

Organization

Where the environmental assessment is external in nature, the organization assessment is more internally focused. One way of thinking about this is through the use of a SWOT analysis (strengths, weaknesses, opportunities, and threats). What are your internal capacities and capabilities?

Culture

Organizational culture has a distinct impact on which design is chosen. We have previously described *culture* as that system of shared norms, beliefs, and behaviors that govern the activities of the members of the group. One of the important things to keep in mind is that multiple cultures can exist in a single organization—in fact, most organizations are multicultural. The selection and imposition of any organization design must take into account the prevailing cultures. The aspect of culture is particularly important in public health organizations given the fact that public health as a profession embraces diversity in all forms. Simply crafting an organization design based on the dominant culture is antithetical to the principles and practices of public health. Your challenge will be to think through an organization design that respects and supports the cultures of your entire workforce.

Human Resources

Sometimes, we provide human characteristics to inanimate objects, and this is frequently the case with organizations. In fact, without human resources, organizations are nothing but collections of buildings, desks, and technology. Any organization design must take into account the people who will be asked to populate the new parts of the organization.

Politics

One of the important things for public health leaders to keep in mind is the political attributes of their organization. While there may be formal structures, reporting relationships, and methods, there are frequently distinct political realities that mediate organizational effectiveness. Any organization design must take into account the politics in place at that moment.

Forms of Organization Design

Now that the public health leader has in mind the core principles of organization design or redesign and has gone through the factors influencing the selection of design, now it is time to think about the specific form that might be put into place. The work by Charnes and Tewksbury (1993) is most helpful in this regard. They posit that there are five organization designs of increasing level of integration by program. The five designs are functional, divisional, matrix, parallel, and program.

Functional

Take a look at almost any organization chart and you will see a functional form of organization design. There is a clear linear hierarchy of departments and reporting relationships. It is clear who reports to whom, and information flow is clearly defined. Functional organization designs are generally most appropriate in environments that are stable and predictable.

Divisional

In more complex organizations, it makes sense to group functions around divisions, each of which is responsible for its own administrative operations. This allows for a significant level of autonomy on the part of each division, but, at the same time, certain resources can be provided centrally such as information services, payroll, and purchasing of supplies. This is a complex form and requires significant coordination between and among divisions, particularly with respect to making sure that everyone is working to improve overall organizational function and not just that of his or her particular division.

Matrix

Matrix organizations became popular a number of years ago in an attempt to overcome the problems of functional and divisional designs. In this case, functional and program or product line managers are jointly responsible for specific activities. In the case of our county health department, there might be program managers around water quality, immunizations, and infectious disease and then functional managers for the areas of nursing, finance, government relations, and others. These managers would then interact with one another on multiple activities. One clear concern with matrix organizations is that workers below the managerial level have two bosses instead of just one. It can also be expensive in terms of personnel costs and multiple accountability systems.

Parallel

In parallel designs, the ideal state is to allow persons to better manage and respond to both internal and external environmental changes. In health care, this design is most clearly seen in the recent growth of quality improvement (QI) efforts. Many organizations have developed quality councils that run parallel to the larger organization and function to identify areas where QI measures can be put into place and improvements made in client services. Some of the places QI activities might be used include reducing client waiting times to see a clinician, identifying and reducing staff turnover in a particular department, or improving access to community mental health services. QI teams are formed by pulling representatives from across the organization regardless of their place in the hierarchy. The idea is to get those persons closest to the work itself focused on improving how work is done because they are the ones who truly know what they are doing. Given the acceptance of QI by various public and private accreditation bodies, this type of organization design serves to make QI an organization norm rather than just another task. The downside to this design is that it takes significant personnel time to be part of the meetings, can divert attention from routine work that still needs to be accomplished, and may cause conflict over priorities.

Program

Program design (sometimes called product/service line management) places a single person in charge of all aspects of a given product/service or group of products/services. This person is in charge of coordinating all aspects of budgets, personnel, marketing, and other functional resources for their product or service. Among the advantages to program design is that redundancies can be identified and eliminated, and marketing strategies to promote the service to the most appropriate group can be put into place. Simply putting a design like this into place is a challenge to many organizations. The right services need to be grouped together, and selecting and training the right product/service line managers can be difficult.

In summary, organization design is a dynamic process that depends on public health leaders who are willing to change the ways they have done things in the past, who are aware of strong and weak signals in their environments, and who have the vision to see the sort of design that is the best fit for the current and near-term conditions of their organization. In public health settings, the choice of organization design is particularly important. Selecting the most appropriate design allows you to best meet the needs of your community and, at the same time, take full advantage of the organizational resources at your disposal.

GOVERNING BOARD RELATIONSHIPS

Before we begin our discussion about the governing board and your relationship with it, it is important to distinguish between *governance* and *management*. Earlier in this book, the roles of the manager were discussed at length. While you have a tremendous level of responsibility for the day-to-day operations of your organization, the legal authority for the organization resides with the governing board and not with you or any of your staff. When the organization is sued in court for injury, damage, or some other civil wrong, the governing board is named as the defendant given it is the legal representative of the organization. In fact, the language that is used is that if you are the CEO (or equivalent), you serve at the pleasure of the governing board. In many cases, the CEO finds that his or her job has been terminated subsequent to the governing board having met the previous evening.

In the public sector, there are three broad classes of boards: honorary, fiduciary, and community. *Honorary boards* (some-times called advisory boards) have no legal standing and exist to provide advice to the executive management team, and (frequently) the members are there because of their financial standing in the community and their willingness to give significant sums of money to the organization. *Fiduciary boards* are those that have the legal responsibility for the functions of the organization and are more carefully discussed later. Their legal authority comes via the articles of incorporation filed when the organization first came into being and the organization's bylaws. These groups may or may not have community representation. *Community boards* are those where the bylaws require a majority of community members as opposed to officers from the organization.

While not as apparent as in for-profit or not-for-profit acute care organizations, the governing board in public health organizations is just as important and requires just as much care as any other entity. In a general sense, the governing board is legally responsible for everything that happens in your organization, and the members of the governing board have a personal and collective fiduciary duty for all aspects of organizational operations. One of the assumptions that we make in this section is that your organization is either a public or not-for-profit entity and not a for-profit one. While the board responsibilities are very similar, there are specific prohibitions associated with your organization that are not present in for-profits. In this section, we examine three vital attributes of the relationship between you and your governing board: roles and responsibilities of the governing board, governing board composition, and managing your relationship with the governing board.

Roles and Responsibilities

Whether it is called a board of directors, governing board, or some other name, the governing board of your organization has the ultimate authority for everything that takes place in the organization. For the purposes of this discussion, we distinguish between general and specific responsibilities for the board. General responsibilities include the following:

- *Governance.* The board is obligated to make sure that the organization is run according to the laws and regulations of the particular state in which it operates. The board has broad oversight responsibilities for anything that takes place in the organization and is potentially liable for any errors, injury, or damage that might occur as a result of the actions of any employee. Board governance is spelled out under the terms of the organization's bylaws and includes information on how board members are selected, terms of office, committee structure, and other critical items.

- *Leadership.* In association with the chief executive officer (or equivalent senior administrator), the board guides the mission and direction of the organization. In most cases, the board is responsible for crafting or amending the organization's strategic plan including the mission, vision, and values.
- *Stewardship.* The board's role is to ensure that any and all funds are used for the benefit of the public. In this role, the board has a central fiduciary duty to use the assets of the organization solely for the benefit of the organization and those who the organization serves. It is never permissible for a board member to gain private inurement or private benefit from serving as a member of the board. This includes a prohibition against any part of the net earnings of the organization from going to a board member or his or her family in the form of salary or other compensation.

There are a limited number of specific roles for the board, including:

- Hiring, evaluating, and (when necessary) terminating the CEO.
- Reviewing and approving the annual budget.
- Reviewing and approving major organizational decisions, commitments, and plans, including expenditures, loans, and leases.
- Evaluating progress toward strategic, programmatic, and financial goals.
- Select members to serve on the board, and evaluate the performance of the board itself.
- Meet on a regularly scheduled basis.
- Update the bylaws as needed.

Governing Board Composition

We mentioned earlier that the legal authority for the governing board resides with the articles of incorporation (filed with the state in which the organization was originally incorporated) and the bylaws. There is no rule dictating how many persons should be on the governing board, but as a general rule of thumb, the larger the board, the more difficult it will be to get members to the meetings and, often, to gain concurrence on important issues. According to BoardSource, the average size of nonprofit boards nationally is 16, although the minimum number is dictated by each state.

The challenge for the leaders of public health organizations is in terms of the actual membership of the board. For leaders of state and county health departments and other public entities, the governing board can be (but is not always) made up of elected officials. These governing boards are typ-

ically much smaller than those of private organizations, although they have the same set of general and specific roles and responsibilities. The most important thing to keep in mind is that for elected officials, your organization is probably not the most important item on their agenda. The odds are that these people are trying to balance competing interests, and (except in a crisis situation) there are probably more pressing interests. As politicians, most are interested in getting reelected and have to be sensitive to the needs and demands of their constituents. The unfortunate truth is that the majority of the public is relatively unaware of the importance of public health, and getting people to agree to increase taxes to fund new services (or maintain existing services) is not something most elected officials care to promote. The other important consideration for this group of governing board members is that serving in this role is but one item on a whole list of other things they have to do, so getting and keeping their attention may be difficult.

The other types of boards frequently encountered include those that are part of private, not-for-profit organizations. The majority of those boards come from the community and are drawn to your organization through some combination of belief in what you are doing, a positive experience with your organization or services provided, a desire to give back to the community, or some combination of these or other reasons. Sometimes, board members are selected because of their history of making major financial gifts to your organization. Your board members will likely have skills in their particular area of expertise but generally not in public health; however, the occasional clinician might join the board. One of the challenges for community-based nonprofit boards is to select members with the sorts of skills and experience that bring added depth and perspective to the board and the organization.

Managing Your Relationship with the Governing Board

As the leader of the public health organization, you serve at the pleasure of the governing board. You are the one and only person the board hires, evaluates, and terminates. Therefore, your relationship with the governing board (your bosses) must be carefully managed for your, as well as your organization's, effectiveness. There are a number of important elements that are part of this relationship:

- *Board education.* Given that most of the board members are well-intentioned and energetic but not educated or experienced in public health, your job will be to educate board members (particularly new members) about the specifics of what your organization does and the important role it has in the community. This educational process must be continuous because you cannot assume that the board has your institutional memory. In addition, words and acronyms that are part of your everyday vocabulary may be completely foreign to your board. Board members need to be clear about their role, duties, and expectations (as we discussed earlier). Some organizations have a lengthy manual for new board members or actually send them to training.

- *Communication.* Understanding that there is a structure to the board (including a chair and an executive committee), your job is to clearly communicate to the entire board. The idea of redundant communication was mentioned earlier in this chapter and is particularly important here. The executive committee is a very small subset of the board that is sometimes, but not always, made up of the chair, chair-elect, immediate past chair, and perhaps the heads of a few important subcommittees (such as finance or membership).

- *Listening.* Too often, we assume that communication begins and ends when we have said what we have to say and then it is time to move on. Some of the most effective CEOs take the time to carefully listen to the thoughts and viewpoints of all of their board members. When all is said and done, you want your board to move your organization in the direction you want. This is much more likely to occur if all members feel as though they have been heard and that their opinions are valued.

- *Do more than just give reports.* Board meetings are notorious for receiving reports and little more. Boards that are engaged in subcommittees and have a voice in major decisions are much more likely to better understand the needs of your organization and serve in an advocacy position for you.

- *Respect the time of your board.* As noted earlier, every member of your board has other commitments and is not getting paid for his or her board service. Be sure to respect the time being given by your board members by starting and ending the meetings on time, getting materials to them in a timely manner, and providing a lunch or other form of refreshment (depending on when the meeting is taking place). Above all, be gracious and genuine in thanking your board members individually for their service.

One other important item is the role of the executive session, or the ability of the members of the governing board to go into private session and talk just among themselves. For most board meetings, you and select members of your staff will be in attendance along with guests and interested members from the public. You and certain staff may have voting privileges, depending on the wording of the bylaws. However, particularly when conversations about the subject of your evaluation occur, the board may want to go into executive session. At that time, you and any of your staff will be excused from the meeting. Protocol is that the outcome of that executive session will be discussed with you either verbally or in writing by the chair and/or the executive committee. For most senior leaders, being excused from a board meeting is a nerve-wracking process full of uncertainty. If you have a good relationship with the board, and particularly the chair, you should be aware of why an executive session is being called. As is the case in managing your staff, staff members should be aware of the kind of job you think they are doing before receiving their performance evaluation. The same thing should hold for your evaluation.

It should be noted that there is a recent trend for boards to go into more frequent executive sessions, with the idea that it can talk more openly and candidly about organizational importance when the executive is not there. While this might be the stated reason, one of the reasons might be that the board is experiencing a lack of trust in the executive. Should your board be going into executive session more frequently than normal, you should find the time to have a frank and open conversation with the chair about your relationship with the board.

CONCLUSION

Public health organizations have always been made to work under conditions of severe resource constraints. Yet historically, the focus on the mission and overarching goals of improving the health of the public has kept these organizations moving forward, despite the challenge of sometimes inadequate funding and lack of public support. Creating high levels of organizational effectiveness are more important today than ever before. This chapter examined three critical attributes of highly effective public health organizations: team building, organization design, and relationship with the governing board. Leaders of public health organizations of all sorts must be adaptable in all three areas. While funding will never be completely adequate, your duty calls for you to make the most out of the human, financial, technological, and other resources at your disposal. Under the best of circumstances, this is a challenging time to be in a leadership position in public health, but by making the most of your resources, you can more effectively fulfill your critical mission and meet the needs of your community.

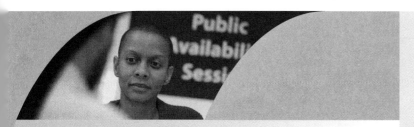

Discussion Questions

1. What appear to be the characteristics of effective teams in public health settings? What roles do managers play in facilitating the work of those teams?

2. Suppose for a minute that you have a staff member who is well-known, is highly productive, and is highly respected by his or her peers. However, he or she is also known as having a disruptive personality, and several staff members have come to you to complain about how demeaningly this person treats them. How will you handle this person?

3. Distinguish among the five broad forms of organization design. Where might you find examples of each one of them in public heath settings?

4. What are the core duties of the governing board of a public health organization? Given that, in many cases, the governing board is made up of elected officials and its composition is totally out of the control of the administrator, how can public health leaders help shape decisions made by the governing board?

5. Distinguish between management and leadership. Can managers engage in leadership activities? How? Do leaders also have management duties? Please explain.

REFERENCES

Albanese R, Van Fleet DD. Rational behavior in groups: The free riding tendency. *Academy of Management Review.* 1985;10:244–255.

Bales RF. Interaction Process Analysis. Cambridge, MA: Addison-Wesley; 1950.

Charnes M, Smith-Tewksbury LJ. *Collaborative Management in Health Care.* San Francisco: Jossey-Bass; 1993.

Etzioni A. *A comparative analysis of complex organizations.* New York: Free Press; 1961.

Fried BJ, Topping S, Edmondson AC. Groups and teams. In: *Health Care Management: Organization Design and Behavior.* 5th ed. Clifton Park, NY: Thompson Delmar Learning; 2006.

Hackman JR. Introduction. Work teams in organizations. An orienting framework. In: Hackman JR, ed. *Groups That Work (And Those That Don't):* *Creating Conditions for Effective Teamwork.* San Francisco: Jossey-Bass; 1990.

Owens DA, Mannic EA, Neale MA. Strategic formation of groups: Issues in task performance and team member selection. In Gruenfeld DH, ed. *Research on Managing Groups and Teams.* Stamford, CT: MAI Press; 1998:149–165.

Hackman JR. Work design. In Hackman JR, Suttle JL, eds. *Improving Work Life at Work.* Santa Monica, CA: Goodyear; 1976.

Janis L. *Victims of Groupthink.* Boston: Houghton-Mifflin; 1972.

Mintzberg H. *Structures in Fives: Designing Effective Organizations.* Englewood Cliffs, NJ: Prentice-Hall; 1983.

Tuckman BW. Developmental sequences in small groups. *Psychological Bulletin.* 1965;63:384–399.

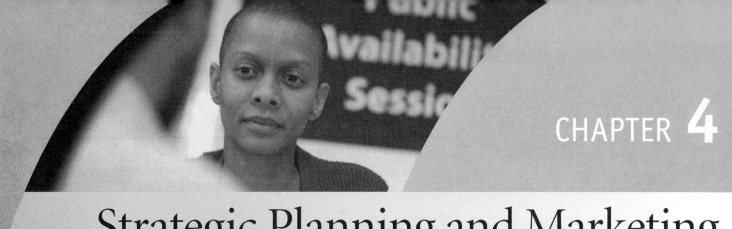

CHAPTER 4

Strategic Planning and Marketing for Public Health Managers

Leonard H. Friedman

"Cheshire Puss . . . would you tell me, please, which way I go from here?"
"That depends a good deal on where you want to get to," said the Cat.
"I don't much care where—" said Alice.
"Then it doesn't much matter which way you go," said the Cat.
"—so long as I get somewhere," Alice added as an explanation.
"Oh, you're sure to do that," said the Cat. (Carroll, 1960)

INTRODUCTION

The idea of marketing and strategic planning for public health managers might, on the surface, appear to be counterintuitive. After all, unlike most other goods and services, the products and activities generated by public health organizations are not bought and sold on the open market. While you must maintain an adequate cash flow in order to pay your staff, purchase supplies, and pay your utility bill, the people in the communities you serve are not actually paying for most of what you actually provide. You may compete for contracts and grants in order to make a special project available, but most of your activities are provided to clients for little if any direct cost to them. Taking the time to develop long-term plans and strategies might appear to be a waste of your valuable time and energy, particularly considering all of the things that your organization is obligated to provide.

In actual fact, marketing and strategic planning are essential skills for each and every public health manager. You want people to know what you do and to use your services. You probably want to project a positive image to current and future clients. You definitely need to build an organization that attracts and retains outstanding staff, even if you cannot necessarily pay them what they might earn in the private sector. Despite the pressure of clients and community members for more and more services, you need to make difficult decisions about the actual needs of the community and what it is you can actually provide.

LEARNING OBJECTIVES

After reading this chapter, the reader will be able to:

1. Determine and articulate the linkage of an organization's mission, vision, and values to its strategic direction.
2. Choose from among several analytic tools to help determine strategic choice.
3. Perform a SWOT (strength, weakness, opportunity, threat) analysis to evaluate the internal and external organizational environment.
4. Articulate strategies that are in alignment with the social and cultural assets and expectations of diverse cultures and communities.

TOPIC PRESENTATION

A very wise man once said, "Life is choice." This idea applies to organizations just as neatly as it does to individuals. We have choices to make on multiple levels. In most cases, the choices are relatively minor and inconsequential. Shall I have chicken or fish for dinner tonight? Will I take a walk or read a book? Other personal decisions are much larger in scope and have a far greater long-term impact. Where should I to go to college, and what should I study? Who shall I marry, and will we have children? There are different thought processes that go into each type of decision. The former usually require relatively little forethought and planning, whereas the later typically demand that the decision maker think through multiple pathways to the decision, the long-term impact the decision might have, alternatives that might be equally attractive, and the costs associated with moving forward on the decision.

Organizations do very similar things when considering decisions that need to be made by persons in leadership roles. There are countless numbers of small decisions that must be made daily to keep an organization moving forward. Who will be working this week? Should we schedule the delivery of supplies today or tomorrow? What color will the reception area be painted? Other organizational decisions are neither simple nor easy to make. What type of service needs to be offered to best meet the needs of our community? Should we discontinue offering a program that few clients use but that has been part of our organization since the beginning? Do we need to restructure our organization to better cope with the severe downturn in the economy?

These examples of organizational decisions fall under the heading of *strategic decisions*. Prior to making decisions like these, public health leaders need significant amounts of real-time data and must carefully weigh the alternatives, consider the consequences of acting and not acting, and think through the financial and personnel implications of any decision. To make the best possible decisions, public health leaders must engage in a process of deliberate strategic thinking. For our purposes, we define *strategic thinking* as an individual intellectual process, a mindset, or a method of intellectual analysis that asks people to position themselves as leaders and see the "big picture." Vision and a sense of the future are an inherent part of strategic thinking but at the same time strategic thinkers draw upon the past, understand the present, and envision an improved future (Swayne, Duncan, & Ginter, 2006, p. 19). The best strategic thinkers accept change as absolutely necessary, understand the causes and results of change, and continually work to craft an intentional future for their organization based on change. Strategic thinkers:

- Acknowledge the reality of change.
- Question current assumptions and realities.
- Build an understanding of systems.
- Envision possible futures.
- Generate new ideas.
- Consider the fit of their organization with the external environment (Swayne et al., 2006, p. 19).

At this point, it should be clear that strategic thinking is a necessary but not sufficient condition. Thinking needs to be coupled with action. Yet, as a prelude to action, we need to plan. In this case, *strategic planning* is the periodic process of developing a set of steps for an organization to accomplish its mission and vision by using strategic thinking (Swayne et al., 2006, p. 21). When done properly, strategic planning yields the following:

- Provides a sequential, step-by-step process for creating a strategy.
- Involves periodic brainstorming sessions.
- Requires data and information, but also builds in consensus and judgment.

- Establishes an organizational focus.
- Facilitates consistent decision-making processes.
- Reaches consensus on what is required to help the organization fit with the external environment.
- Results in a documented strategic plan.

Coupling strategic thinking and strategic planning is particularly important for public health leaders. It will come as no surprise to any of you that you have a long list of required tasks and frequently inadequate resources to accomplish your mission. According to the Centers for Disease Control and Prevention and the Office of the Chief of Public Health Practice, there are 10 essential public health services that define the responsibilities of local public health systems:

1. Monitor health status to identify and solve community health problems.
2. Diagnose and investigate health problems and health hazards in the community.
3. Inform, educate, and empower people about health issues.
4. Mobilize community partnerships and action to identify and solve health problems.
5. Develop policies and plans that support individual and community health efforts.
6. Enforce laws and regulations that protect health and ensure safety.
7. Link people to needed personal health services and ensure the provision of health care when otherwise unavailable.
8. Ensure a competent public and personal healthcare workforce.
9. Evaluate effectiveness, accessibility, and quality of personal and population-based health services.
10. Research for new insights and innovative solutions to health problems.

This is a long and impressive list. Which are the most critical to your local community? Do you have the resources needed to carry out each part equally well? What is happening in your community and beyond that might affect both the demand for related services and your ability to provide them? To begin to answer these questions, we must start with a careful examination of our external and internal environments.

ENVIRONMENTAL ASSESSMENT

External Environmental Analysis

All of us and all of our organizations are profoundly affected by our external environments. Think for a moment about someone who sails. While the desired outcome is straightforward (I wish to go from point A to point B), the process is highly dependent on the external environment, specifically wind and current. The successful sailor knows how to read these strong and weak signals found in the external environment and then use them to his or her advantage. Astute public health leaders do the same thing, but in this case, it is worthwhile to find a way to help guide their organizations toward an intended goal. There are a number of important objectives for understanding and analyzing the external environment:

- Categorize and evaluate important issues that will affect the organization.
- Think through how outside organizations will affect the public health entity.
- Assess both strong and weak signals from emerging issues that can affect the organization.
- Speculate on future issues and the changes they might have on the organization.
- Provide organized information that will help strategic planning throughout the organization.

The external environment is so vast that public health leaders need a way to make sense of how the environment is structured and how to evaluate the changes that are continually taking place. For public health organizations, the external environment is populated with a number of important stakeholders including (but not limited to):

- Government institutions.
- Business organizations.
- Educational institutions.
- Religious organizations.
- Foundations and research institutions.
- Individuals and families.

While it is necessary and important to know the many parts of the external environment, it is just as important to be able to analyze what is happening outside of your organization in a coherent and meaningful way. There are four steps to this analysis: (1) environmental scanning, (2) issue monitoring, (3) forecasting of future issues, and (4) issue assessment.

Environmental Scanning

So much raw data are available in the external environment that there needs to be a way of systematically looking at information. Keep in mind that there are multiple sources of data and information, including news media, professional meetings, government reports, and meeting minutes, to name a few. There needs to be a way to categorize and make sense of all these data. One good way of doing that is to categorize the data into several different "boxes," such as technological, political, economic, social, and regulatory. The job of the public health leader is to make sure that the environment is contin-

ually scanned for changes in each of these areas and that the most current data are available for use by decision leaders.

Issue Monitoring

Tracking trends, issues, and events that have been identified through the scanning process is part of issue monitoring. More than just continually scanning the environment for changes, issue monitoring looks to build up a database around a particular issue. An example of this in public health might be avian flu and changes that are taking place overseas in terms of the incidence and prevalence of the disease.

Forecasting of Future Issues

Public health leaders must try to answer the question, "If these trends continue or accelerate beyond their present rate, what will the issue look like in the future and how might we be affected?" Using the avian flu example, issue forecasting might ask how the public health agency might respond should the disease reach epidemic proportions in their local area.

Issue Assessment

Issue assessment attempts to assess the effect that the expected change in the environment will have on the organization. This is particularly difficult given that issue monitoring and forecasting involve "what if" scenarios. Let us return to our avian flu case. We can predict with only minimal certainty what affect a severe outbreak would have on a given community. Computer models might be available to help in the process, but ultimately, it is the experience and judgment of public health leaders that make sense out of unclear, ambiguous, and often conflicting data.

Case Example

You are employed as the Director of the Infectious Disease Office of your state health department. You depend on your small staff to help collect information from multiple outside sources about disease outbreaks. Most of your work is pretty routine and centers around spikes in measles in children or the all-too-frequent hepatitis A reports from persons who ate at restaurants where employees did not properly wash their hands. However, today as you were driving into work you heard a radio interview with an emergency room physician in your state, who told the reporter that she had no idea why there seemed to be an unusual number of persons who appeared in her ER in severe respiratory distress. You have seen no e-mails nor received any faxes about anything unusual. How might you deal with this new information?

Internal Environmental Analysis and Value Creation

Developing a full and complete understanding of the external environment is critical for any organization. However, this is only part of the picture. It is just as important for public health leaders to have an equally full and complete understanding of their internal environment. What are the systems and subsystems available to help the organization fulfill its mission and meet the needs of its clients? How do you evaluate your activities, including clinical operations, human resources, information systems, administrative management, and so on? Stated another way, how and where do you bring value to your clients and community? Building from the work of Michael Porter (1985), we can imagine the value created by public health organizations as determined by the services that are delivered and the activities that support service delivery.

Service delivery activities (the actual process of making public health services available to client groups) can be divided into pre-service, point-of-service, and after-service. Let us imagine that you wish to set up an immunization clinic for school-age children in a way that is caring and convenient for everyone in the community. There are a number of pre-service activities you might consider. What are the demographics of your community? Is there a high demand for immunizations? Is there a way to offer this service that is convenient for most consumers? Can this service be advertised in local media? What will you charge for the shots? Will appointments be needed, or can you do this on a walk-in basis?

Once the client arrives, the point-of-service activities begin. Is the environment neat and clean? Is the paperwork available in adequate quantity, and is translation service available if needed? Is there minimal waiting time? Is the caregiver courteous, and does he or she ease the stress to both the child and the parent? Is adequate information about side effects given?

Your clinic can create value by the after-care processes. How is payment processed? A short telephone call the next day to make sure that there are no unexpected side effects is a wonderful idea.

The other half of value creation is through the various support activities that your organization provides and includes organization culture, organization structure, and strategic resources—all of which are designed to aid in the efficient and effective delivery of services. While clients may never see these things, all of them act to either help or hinder the ability of staff to do their best work.

In order to complete your internal environmental analysis, we recommend a three-step process: (1) identify internal strengths and weaknesses, (2) evaluate your relevance in the community, and (3) focus on strengths.

Identify Internal Strengths and Weaknesses

This is an absolutely essential part of any strategic assessment. You must identify those things that your organization does well and those that you do poorly. One method that is frequently used is a SWOT analysis. Public health leaders and their teams should sit down and think through internal *strengths* and *weaknesses* along with external *opportunities* and *threats*. Ask yourself which of those things you identify as strengths and weaknesses are relative or absolute. Relative strengths and weaknesses have to be measured against the ability of others in your environment to do the same thing. How well does the local private hospital or physician clinic provide the same sorts of clinical services as you? Absolute (or objective) strengths and weaknesses are those that are clear and cannot easily be changed. Part of the identification of strengths and weaknesses is your ability to assess the capacity and capability of your organization to deliver the services required. Do you have adequate numbers of properly trained staff? Do you possess the level of technology necessary to do the job? Are you overwhelmed doing other required tasks and are now being asked to do something entirely different?

Evaluate Your Relevance in the Community

The fact is that for many things you do, there are others in your community who do the same thing and are competing with you for revenue, prestige, and stature. While public health organizations are frequently mandated to perform certain activities that are required by statute, there are other roles in which you do compete with the private sector. In those areas, you need to think about the following questions:

- *Value.* Is what you do seen as valuable to current or future customers?
- *Rareness.* Are you the only group that does what you do, or are there others who have similar resources, competencies, and capabilities?
- *Imitability.* Is it easy or difficult to duplicate what you do or provide?
- *Sustainability.* Can what you do or provide be maintained over time? (Swayne et al., 2006, p. 169)

Focus on Strengths

It is at this point that you have to honestly assess where you stack up against others in your service area that provide similar services to you. The question you need to answer is why you are either continuing to or planning to provide services in areas in which you are not strong. Given that all organizations have specific strengths, you need to identify those and not try to be someone you are not.

STRATEGIC CHOICE

Having conducted a thorough external and internal environmental assessment, it is now time to think about the choice of strategy. Actually, strategic choice is limited to three main options: you can grow, contract, or stay the same. The role of the public health leader is to determine which combination of these options to employ. Rather than rushing into choosing one or another strategic option, we recommend that you employ a deliberative and thoughtful process that begins with a consideration of your organization's mission, vision, and values.

Mission, Vision, and Values

Every important strategic decision that an organization makes must be aligned with its mission, vision, and values. Public health organizations are no exception. A strategy that is not derived from the mission, vision, and values is without a clear path and may actually be counterproductive to the organization and the community it serves.

Mission

A well-written mission statement speaks clearly to the distinctiveness of the organization. It is an enduring statement of purpose that is broadly defined. The mission statement identifies the scope of operations of the organization as well as the market served. Take, for example, the mission statement from Boulder County Public Health:

> Boulder County Public Health shall protect, promote, and enhance the health and well-being of all people and the environment in Boulder County.

This brief and well-written mission statement tells the reader what Boulder County Public Health does and the market they serve.

Another example of a mission statement is from the Michigan Department of Community Health, Office of Public Health Preparedness:

> The Office of Public Health Preparedness (OPHP) in the Michigan Department of Community Health is charged with protecting the health of Michigan citizens against chemical, biological, and radiological threats. OPHP focuses on minimizing the threat to health from terrorist acts, accidents, and other incidents. We collaborate with local, state, and federal authorities to stay ahead of forces that threaten the health of Michigan citizens.

In this case, it is clear to the community and the staff exactly what the OPHP is and what they do. You know their target market and the geographic area in which they operate.

Finally, let us look at one more mission statement, this time from the Lourdes Health System Center for Public Health:

> The Lourdes Center for Public Health works collaboratively with academic and community partners to identify critical public health challenges, design and implement research, and develop intervention strategies for urban and vulnerable populations. The Center's focus is to utilize research findings to provide immediate benefits to communities, reduce health care disparities, and foster public health care quality improvement.

This mission statement speaks to uniqueness of the organization and clearly identifies the scope of operations in terms of the services they provide. In addition, the Lourdes Center for Public Health makes clear its key stakeholders. Notice that in all cases, the mission statement is concise and satisfies the test of being able to fit on the back of a business card.

Vision

If the mission tells staff and clients who the organization is and what they do, then the vision seeks to describe what the organization wishes to become and its hope for the future. According to Swayne and colleagues (2006), well-written vision statements have the following attributes:

- Are inspiring and potentially revolutionary.
- Are clear, challenging, and focused on excellence.
- Make sense to the key stakeholders and, at the same time, are flexible.
- Are stable but changed when necessary.
- Provide a clear sense of direction.
- Empower staff and employees first.
- Prepare for the future while honoring the past.
- Lead to tangible results.

Pulling it all together, let us look some examples of vision statements taken from various public health organizations and ask how they compare to the attributes just mentioned.

> The vision of the Western New York Public Health Alliance is to improve the health, safety, and wellness of our eight-county region.
> Mental Health America envisions a just, humane, and healthy society in which all people are accorded respect, dignity, and the opportunity to achieve their full potential through meaningful social inclusion that is free from discrimination.
> A city with a vision will remain constantly alive and responsive to the welfare of its people.

We, the (Berkeley, CA) Health and Human Services Department, will continue to be an essential resource, working in partnership with the community to enrich its future. We envision a city:

- Where diversity is valued, acknowledged and respected;
- Where people thrive and realize their fullest potential;
- Where there is individual and collective responsibility for maintaining a safe and healthy environment;
- Where the resources of our city are maximized and invested in the best interests of the community;
- Where there is community collaboration to establish prevention-focused public policy for the common good;
- Where citizens and staff are truly valued, nurtured, and respected for their essential contributions to the community;
- Where people respect mutual differences and seek common ground;
- Where norms are challenged and people take risks to create meaningful and innovative change;
- Where everyone has a place to call home; and
- Where people have a birthright to a hopeful future.

Values

Values are the core principles that organizations and the people within them stand for and that serve to make the organization unique. In many corporate settings, you will see values that include language about ethics and ethical behavior. Because ethical behavior is rarely a problem in public health settings, you might see a very different set of values, as noted in the following examples:

Arlington, Virginia, Public Health Services

- Quality healthcare and community services, including mental health and substance abuse, accessible and affordable to all.
- Services provided in the least restrictive environment for the consumer.
- Utilizing community health resources effectively by focusing on prevention as much as treatment.
- A healthy lifestyle that emphasizes good nutrition and physical activity, through support of health education

programs and community activities accessible to all members.

- Community input and adapting services and infrastructure to meet the community's changing needs.
- Learning as a lifelong process, where each individual has the opportunity to live life to his or her fullest potential.
- A welcoming community where each member has a voice and feels a sense of belonging, recognizing the diversity of its members.
- Personal and community safety as a right and a shared responsibility so that all who live, work, and play here can pursue healthy activities.
- A prepared community that anticipates and responds quickly to protect the safety and welfare of its members.
- High-quality air, water, public spaces, and other environmental resources.
- Strong partnerships with businesses, organizations, universities, and others to promote economic vitality.

Dane County (WI) Department of Human Services

- All people have value.
- All will be treated with respect, dignity, and confidentiality.
- Diversity strengthens our community.
- We promote individual and family independence.
- We strive to provide efficient, effective, and accessible services.
- We support collaboration and the integration of services.
- We promote prevention, early intervention, and rehabilitation.
- We value new and innovative approaches to providing services.
- We manage public funds responsibly.
- We promote community-based services in the least restrictive setting.

Strategic Goals

Taken together, the mission, vision, and values of an organization provide the focus and direction for the choice of strategic goals. These goals then become the foundation for the strategic plan. The best-written strategic goals have the following attributes:

- They should relate specifically to attributes critical to accomplishing the mission.
- They should connect critical success factors and the momentum needed to carry out specific objectives.

- They should be limited in number with a focus on the critical few rather than the trivial many.
- They should be crafted by leaders but stated in terms that everyone in the organization can understand.

Strategic Alternatives

Now that the mission, vision, values, and strategic goals have been crafted, it is time for the decision makers to come up with their choice of strategic alternatives. No matter which alternative is selected, it must satisfy the following criteria: address an important external issue; build on the strength of the organization or help correct a weakness; align with mission, vision, and values; move the organization toward achieving the vision; and achieve one or more strategic goals.

There are three overarching strategic alternatives: growth, contraction, or maintenance (sometimes called status quo). *Growth strategies* are chosen when you have identified an unmet need in your community that you can successfully address. The primary growth strategies include those that allow you to diversify into new products or services in new markets, offer current products or services to new markets, offer new products or services in existing markets, and grow products or services in existing markets. *Contraction strategies* serve to reduce the number of services that the organization offers. This can be done by selling off all or part of a particular service unit, selling the assets of an organization or perhaps shrinking the size of a market, or reducing the services that are made available to a community. *Maintenance strategies* are used either when current strategies are adequate or the environment is so unstable that it becomes almost impossible to judge what the future might hold. In this case, a public health organization can choose either to retain the status quo or work to incrementally do current things better.

The three primary strategic alternatives are easy to understand and make good sense to all types of organizations. The hard part comes when you, as a leader in your organization, must choose which strategy to use. Selection of the wrong strategy can have devas-

tating consequences for your community and your organization in terms of wasted resources, provision of unwanted or unneeded services, and possible reductions in funding from either private or government sources. How do you choose which strategic alternative to put into place? The fact is that there is never one best choice—rather, there is a range of options, and your job is to evaluate the available data and use that data to help drive your decision. For this discussion, two methods are presented to assess and help decide upon strategic alternatives: the SWOT matrix, and program evaluation.

SWOT Matrix

Earlier in this chapter, we talked about the SWOT analysis as a method by which organizations can systematically evaluate their internal strengths and weaknesses in addition to their external opportunities and threats. Using these data, the public health leader constructs a simple 2 × 2 matrix similar to the one shown in **Table 4-1**.

The internal strengths and weaknesses are listed horizontally and the external opportunities and threats are listed vertically. The decision maker then looks at the list of each variable and determines which is stronger and of greater influence. Based on that evaluation, there are four alternatives:

1. *Survival quadrant.* In this case, internal weaknesses and external threats are the dominant feature. Depending

TABLE 4-1 SWOT Matrix

	Internal Strengths 1. 2. 3. 4.	Internal Weaknesses 1. 2. 3. 4.
External Opportunities 1. 2. 3. 4.	4 Future Quadrant • Growth	2 Internal Fix-It Quadrant • Growth • Maintenance
External Threats 1. 2. 3. 4.	3 External Fix-It Quadrant • Growth • Maintenance	1 Survival Quadrant • Contraction

on the seriousness of the weaknesses and threats, the organization may decide to shut down portions of its operation rather than fund an activity for which there is no support or interest. An example might be an immunization project that had been grant-funded that is no longer supported; in addition, private providers are charging for the same service. Your decision might well be to discontinue the service despite a small need in your community.

2. *Internal fix-it quadrant.* In this situation, there are serious internal weaknesses, but there exist important external opportunities. The presence of external opportunities allows you to try out new services or potentially enter new markets, assuming that your internal weaknesses can be addressed.

3. *External fix-it quadrant.* In this case, there are serious external threats, but the internal strengths are strong and impressive. The presence of significant internal strengths allows you to overcome any threats in the environment. This combination makes it possible for you to offer new products or to enter new markets.

4. *Future quadrant.* In this quadrant, the internal environment is strong, and there are significant external opportunities. In this case, any growth or expansion strategy should work, given that you have the internal capacity and capability and that environmental opportunities outnumber threats.

The SWOT matrix has a number of readily apparent advantages and disadvantages. Among the important advantages are that the analysis is quick and fast to perform, requires few if any resources, and can be done using information that has been previously gathered. The disadvantages of the SWOT matrix are that the analysis is only as good as the data used to prepare it. There is the likelihood that there could be missing or incomplete information, false assumptions might be made, or decisions arrived at quickly with the input of a small number of sources. Despite this, a SWOT matrix is a good tool and should be used as a first step to give guidance as the public health decision leader thinks about the next step in the process.

Program Evaluation

Swayne and colleagues (2006) suggest that public health programs ask themselves the following question: "Does our current set of programs effectively and efficiently fulfill our mission and vision for the future?" In addition, a follow-up question should probably be asked: "Does our public health program have the capacity and capability to provide the breadth of programs that are currently offered?" To make this

determination, it is recommended that public health leaders conduct a needs/capacity analysis and program priority setting via a Q-sort methodology.

The needs/capacity analysis looks very much like a SWOT matrix. Horizontally, we provide an assessment of the organization's capacity to initiate, maintain, and enhance its overall strategy in terms of funding, organizational resources, and skills, and the program's fit with the mission, vision, and values. Vertically, we indicate community needs, including specific requirements for public health services, the availability of services from other public or private sources, and the public/community health objectives. If organizational capacity and community needs are high, then virtually any growth or expansion strategy will work. Similarly, if organizational capacity and community needs are low, then it is time to contract. When organizational capacity is low and community needs are high, it makes sense to maintain what you are doing or perhaps selectively pull out of programs where you cannot effectively meet the need. Finally, if organizational capacity is high but community needs are low, it also makes sense to maintain the status quo or perhaps begin to offer select new services to new markets.

The advantages and disadvantages of the needs/capacity analysis are similar to the SWOT matrix. This is an informative analysis that requires comparatively little data outside of the decision maker's assessment of both the internal and external environments. The disadvantages are also the same in that there is a good likelihood that without good, real-time data you could be drawing the wrong conclusions.

Program priority setting is recommended to public health leaders simply because there is far too much to do with far too little time or resources. Decisions have to be made about what programs and services to support, given the conflicting demands brought about by legal requirements and the specific needs of individuals and groups in the community. The question for the organization is which programs are essential, which are highly desired, and which ones (while good) are not mission-critical. This is particularly important in an environment where resources are scarce and the culture of the organization has been to take on far more than it can actually do with the personnel and financial resources at its disposal. One way of setting program priorities is to get the key organizational stakeholders to reach consensus on what needs to be done first, second, and so on. While this method is certainly democratic, it is cumbersome, time-consuming, and frequently dependent on individual personalities and their ability to support a particular program.

As an alternative, Swayne and her colleagues (2006) recommend the use of the Q-sort method. Q-sort is a ranking process that forces choices where the difference between or among the choices can be very small. In doing a Q-sort, each program that the organization offers is written down on a card. Each member of the management team is then asked to place the cards in a rank order from the most important to the least important. Nine categories are established, with the idea that a normal or quasi-normal distribution of programs will result. One outcome is that the first three categories of programs will be considered for expansion, the second three will stay status quo, and the final three will be considered for contraction. Use of the Q-sort method to set program priorities allows the public health leader to help obtain the opinions of a wide number of stakeholders in a reasonable period of time.

Strategy and Organizational Culture

Organizational culture represents the implicit, invisible, intrinsic, and informal consciousness of the organization that guides the behavior of individuals and shapes itself out of their behavior. Every organization possesses a culture that is knowable to all but is unwritten in any policy or procedure manual. The culture of a public health organization is made up of shared assumptions, shared values, and shared behavioral norms. The *shared assumptions* speak to the things that, as a group, members of the organization are trying to accomplish together. Frequently, these assumptions are expressed in the mission statement. *Shared values* are the way things are done in a particular organization. One thing that should be noted is that the stated values of an organization are frequently different from the actual way things are done. *Shared behavioral norms* are the actions of a group that come about from the activities of the members of the group and are influenced by the informal and frequently unspoken expectations of the members. It should be clear that culture is learned, shared, and both subjective and objective.

So, what does an organization's culture have to do with strategic planning and strategic management? In a culture that encourages staff to take measured risks, there is a much stronger likelihood of innovation and acceptance of change in contrast to a culture that is extremely risk adverse and cautious. At the same time, very cohesive cultures that seem positive and supportive of the members frequently resist change because the members understand that "this is the way we do things around here." New ideas and exciting new directions are frequently discouraged or even dismissed in strong and cohesive cultures. The creation of an organizational strategy embodies a level of change that depends on the type of strategy being enacted. A decision to maintain status quo is the least organizationally disruptive of any strategic decision. An expansion strategy—particularly one offering a new product or service—can create a high level of change if it means bringing on new staff and new ways of doing things. Similarly, contraction strategies can also create a high level of change as familiar and long-held beliefs about services and programs are dismissed when the program is reduced or totally discontinued. The ability of an organization's culture to adapt to change can be one of the most important attributes that allows the public health organization to successfully integrate the new strategy.

CHANGE MANAGEMENT

Think about the ways that you deal with change. How do you like it when change is imposed on you by some outside individual or group and you have little or no input into the process? Imagine further that what is being changed is the way you have done something for a number of years, particularly if you are rather good at it. According to Sirkin, Keenan, and Jackson (2005), there are four attributes that specifically determine the outcome of any change process:

- *Duration*—the length of time needed until a change process is completed.
- *Integrity*—the ability of the team to complete the change process on time.
- *Commitment*—the extent to which senior management is committed to change.
- *Effort*—the amount of time that the change process demands over and above the usual work that still needs to get done.

It should be clear that change management is innately a human process, and those organizations successful at driving change understand that the emotions and feelings of those affected are as important as the specific tasks and outcomes associated with the new way of doing things. In a lengthy article by Goes and colleagues (2000), organizational change is seen as taking place along three dimensions:

- *Level of change.* This is the place where change occurs. Change can take place at the individual, department, or organization level.
- *Frequency of change.* This refers to incremental or continuous change. In most cases, people deal better when there is a break between change processes. Failure to do so can result in a significant level of change fatigue.
- *Control of change.* Most people deal better with change when they have control of the change process (something the authors refer to as "voluntary"). However, a large number of change processes are referred to as deterministic or driven by some external force. An example

of this is the Health Insurance Portability and Accountability Act (HIPAA) regulations that all healthcare organizations need to conform to and have no choice regarding whether or not they wish to implement this change.

There are a number of things that the astute public health manager can do to help his or her organization better handle the change processes that inherently come with any sort of new strategy:

- *Identify the need to change.* Why is this particular strategy being implemented, and how will the public health organization and the community served be better off as a result?
- *Redundant communication.* Your role as a leader is to constantly communicate all aspects of the change process to all staff. When you think that you have communicated enough, do it again.
- *Honesty and integrity.* Lay out an honest and realistic timeline for the accomplishment of specific goals and objectives. It is great to hold staff accountable for getting things done, but you must hold yourself to the same standard.
- *Creating a sense of urgency.* This is sometimes referred to as the "burning platform" requirement. Too often, people will not change unless faced with a crisis or a heightened sense of urgency. The job of the leader is to create the conditions such that people understand that they have no choice but to change.

Another way of thinking about how to manage organizational change came about from the work of Kurt Lewin (1951), who coined the phrase "unfreeze-change-refreeze." In the *unfreeze* phase, the role of management is to make staff uncomfortable with the status quo and create the conditions that allow change to take place. During the *change* phase, it is often necessary to provide coaching to individual staff to help them with the transition to new ways of doing things. *Refreezing* is that period in which the new ways of doing things take root and become part of the public health organization's culture.

At some point, you will experience a level of resistance to the strategic change that you are proposing and starting to implement. The reasons for this resistance are varied but can include turf protection, fear of failure or the unknown, resentment, loss of personal control, and any number of other reasonable explanations. All of these are legitimate in the eyes of the person who is resisting, but it is up to the public health leader to help staff members overcome their resistance. To the greatest extent possible, the person leading the change should:

- Determine who must be involved in planning the change, and include him or her in the decision-making process. Err on the side of involving more people rather than fewer. If there is a question as to whether or not a certain person's support will be needed, include that person.
- Ensure that people from all levels of the organization are involved in planning the change process. This means involving the people who are on the front lines as well. It will be these people who will make the change process succeed or fail.
- Consult with employees from the areas affected by the change when determining the steps needed for change.
- Seek input from people at all levels to establish realistic time frames for specific actions.
- When possible, run a test program with a selected work unit, and solicit feedback on what is working well, where the problem areas are, and how to work out any difficulties.
- Publicly recognize any employees whose suggestions are used in the change process.
- Design a mechanism that provides ongoing feedback from employees throughout the change effort. Involved people are an effective barometer of what is working well and what is not. Ask them to suggest improvements (Wynn, 2008).

While these ideas are all worthwhile and must be part of the repertoire of the skilled public health leader, it must be remembered that one or two disgruntled and unhappy staff members should not be allowed to derail a strategic plan or objective after that plan has been carefully vetted with key stakeholder groups. In these cases, you should certainly listen to the objections of the naysayers, but once that has been done and the decision to move ahead has been made, you must not allow those people to hijack your efforts. In this case, it may be necessary to request a transfer to another part of the organization, or as the worst-case scenario, begin the process of terminating their employment. Your fiduciary duty is to the organization and your clients.

CONCLUSION

Strategic planning and the activities accompanying it are integral to all public health leaders. The ability to carefully evaluate the external and internal organizational environment; determine the capacity and capabilities of the organization; craft a workable mission, vision, and values; develop strategic alternatives; and manage organizational change along with resistance to change is something that will make a profound difference to the public health organization and to the community served. Strategic planning is not something reserved for for-profit companies. Rather, this is a skill that is fundamental in all organizations if they hope to retain their relevance, particularly in an environment of diminished resources and conflicting demands.

Public health organizations have a long and distinguished history of providing programs and services to individuals and communities that are totally dependent on the organization's ability to continually meet the needs of these groups. The value of service is central to all public health organizations. Simply wanting to meet the needs of the community is not enough. Public health leaders have to balance demands from multiple stakeholder groups—all of whom demand that their needs be met first—regardless of shortages of your time, workforce, or other resources. A careful and purposeful process of strategic planning allows the wise public health leader to continuously scan the environment for opportunities, evaluate and prioritize current programs and activities, and be in a position to help his or her organization meet and exceed the expectations of staff and community members.

As the Cheshire cat told Alice, if you don't care where you are going, then any direction you take will get you there. Unfortunately, too many public health organizations have operated under the perspective that planning is a waste of time and energy. The activities of such organizations were heavily dictated by those who provided the funding, and these organizations took pride in doing more and more with less and less. That dictum, while noble, cannot be sustained. Truly effective leaders are those who recognize that they must prioritize, do those things that are of highest value to the community, and either terminate or not perform those activities that can be done elsewhere or that have a minimal benefit. These are the hallmarks of true leadership.

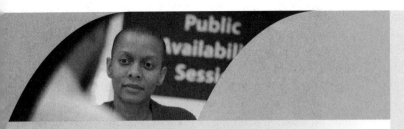

Discussion Questions

1. What is the difference between strategic thinking and strategic planning?

2. List and discuss the elements of a SWOT analysis.

3. Examine the mission, vision, and values statements for your organization. How do they compare with the attributes listed in the chapter?

4. Distinguish among expansion, contraction, and maintenance strategies. How is each type used in public health organizations?

5. One of the frequently used phrases in healthcare management is, "Culture eats strategy for lunch." What do you think that means?

6. Your director has come to you and asked that you take on a new project that will involve a number of large and small changes to the work that your department is currently doing. Provide a brief outline for how you will implement this change.

REFERENCES

Carroll L. *Alice in Wonderland*. New York: Signet Classics; 1960, 1900.

Goes J, Friedman L, Buffa J, Siefert N. A turbulent field: Theory and research on organizational change in health care. *Advances in Healthcare Management*. 2000;1:143–180.

Lewin K. *Field Theory in Social Sciences*. New York: Harper and Row; 1951.

Porter M. *Competitive Advantage: Creating and Sustaining Superior Performance*. New York: Free Press; 1985.

Sirkin H, Keenan P, Jackson A. The hard side of change management. *Harvard Business Review*. 2005;83(10):108–118.

Swayne L, Duncan J, Ginter P. *Strategic Management of Health Care Organizations*. 5th ed. Malden, MA: Blackwell Publishing; 2006.

Wynn G. Change Management. *Managing resistance to change*. Available at: http://managingchange.biz/manage_change_resistance.html. Accessed November 16, 2008.

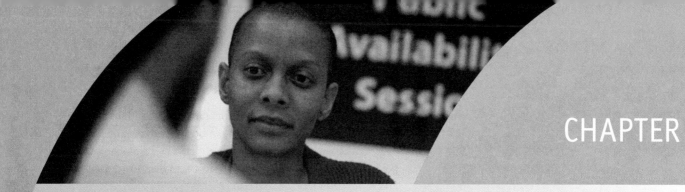

CHAPTER **5**

Conflict Resolution and Negotiation in Healthcare Management

Douglas G. Anderson

"All life is a negotiation."
—Anonymous

INTRODUCTION

Management can be broadly defined as the purposeful interplay of relationships within an organization to achieve defined goals. The success or failure of a manager to achieve these goals can be measured on a number of dimensions, including financial success, realizing measurable outcomes, client or customer satisfaction, and even the continued existence of the organization. But the accomplishment of management activities does not occur in a vacuum of planned and directed action that simply moves from conceived end points to their realization.

The ability to work with and through employees is the benchmark of management. This is especially relevant in healthcare organizations, which are generally more labor-intensive than other industries. And unlike other resources that are utilized to produce services, employees have individual traits and behaviors that can either support or detract from the responsibility of achieving organizational goals. Aligning expectations and performance among employees requires an understanding of the conflicts that inevitably arise from these differences. The effective manager needs a skill set that includes the ability to resolve conflict within an organization.

Organizations are also dependent on external resources for achieving goals. The acquisition of those resources may be a transaction where the manager is precluded from acting independently from market forces. The price set becomes the price taken, and no advantage can be obtained in the transaction. But in many instances, negotiation is possible, and gains for the organization can be obtained by a manager who understands the possibilities of the transaction environment and has the skills to pursue a negotiated advantage. This chapter provides the public health manager with an understanding of both conflict resolution and negotiation in healthcare organizations. Working from theory to specific skills, and through the examination of relevant examples, the manager can learn to develop tools that strengthen the ability to effectively promote organizational goals.

This chapter builds on the chapters addressing management theory. The application of theory in the healthcare environment requires the skillful use of tools to resolve competing interests in the accomplishment of organizational goals. We present a structural context to examine competing interests and provide a framework for success for the public health practitioner.

LEARNING OBJECTIVES

After reading this chapter, the reader will be able to:

1. Describe the reasons that conflict occurs in public health management, and understand the economic, organizational, and psychological bases of conflict in public health organizations.

2. Identify and compare several techniques for conflict management, and apply these techniques in specific examples.

3. Describe several negotiation techniques, and understand the advantages and disadvantages of their utilization in specific situations.

4. Understand the basic factors that affect negotiations, including human behavior, methods of communication, the interactions of negotiation styles, and the type of negotiation being conducted.

5. Identify, design, and modify specific negotiation techniques to resolve conflict and achieve organizational goals in public healthcare management.

CONFLICT RESOLUTION

The Causes of Conflict

The chapter began with the anonymous quote, "All life is a negotiation." Many parents of adolescents will readily agree with this statement. However, in the context of organizational management, this concept incorporates and extends beyond the typical clash of wills that characterizes familial disputes. Conflict in healthcare organizations has many sources: economic, structural, cultural, social, and psychological. The challenge for the public healthcare practitioner is to recognize conflict when it occurs, determine its root causes, and develop effective strategies to resolve the conflict. Consider the following examples of conflict, which typify the challenges of management in healthcare organizations:

- The manager of a community service clinic has two supervisors, each claiming that the other is interfering with staff functions.
- The director of a disaster relief organization is preparing to meet with a major donor to request additional funds to continue the services being provided.
- A medical group practice manager is preparing to meet with an insurance company to request an increase in the reimbursement her organization receives for primary care services.
- The personnel manager in a pubic health department receives a report that a front-desk employee is being rude and uncaring to immigrant families registering for services.
- The supervisor of a small community health center is attempting to evaluate the best deal available in a three-year lease for computers and photocopiers.

Each of these scenarios depicts a conflict that requires effective action by a public health manager to reach a resolution. The sources of these conflicts are varied, and each has implications for both the negotiation strategy that is used to create resolution, as well as the limits of negotiation that confront the manager. The most prominent source of conflict in organizations is derived from a lack of resources. As with all economic activity, public health managers are faced with the basic problem of using scarce resources for competing ends. The application of the concept is most generally recognized in financial terms. Public health managers are constantly in the position of attempting to create healthcare outputs with a limited budget. The reality of resource scarcity is that managers must choose to pursue certain activities and goals and to forego others. This, in turn, creates conflict not only between the overall mission of the organization and its budget, but also among organizational members who require resources to accomplish their responsibilities.

In examining the organization, the public health manager needs to recognize that both organizational structure and management style create sources of conflict. The responsibilities of line managers to accomplish specific activities through subordinate employees are often in conflict with the requirements of staff managers. A typical example is the responsibility delegated in human resources (HR) departments to ensure that personnel are in compliance with applicable state and federal regulations. The HR department requirement to document and orient new hires in Health Insurance Portability and Accountability Act (HIPAA) regulations and Occupational Safety and Health Administration (OSHA) safety procedures can conflict with a nursing supervisor's need to quickly train nurse practitioners to provide well-baby exams in a community clinic. A supervisor who uses an autocratic manner of organizing the work flow in a laboratory setting may create conflict with lab technicians who believe that their knowledge, skills, and abilities entitle them to provide input into departmental work decisions.

Additionally, personal characteristics of employees can also be sources of conflict requiring resolution by the public health manager. Differences in education, religion, gender, communication styles, and individual motivations are all sources of interpersonal conflict within healthcare organizations. For example, the Millennium generation receptionist (born between 1980 and 2001) who has visible tattoos or piercing jewelry may create interpersonal conflict with Baby Boomer secretarial staff, or with clients presenting themselves for clinic services. And in an increasingly diverse country, religious and cultural differences of employees, management, clients, and other significant stakeholders can lead to misunderstandings that constrain the organization from achieving its goals.

Techniques for Conflict Resolution

As the examples demonstrate, there are multiple sources of conflict within the healthcare organization. Conflicts vary widely in their impact in constraining the goals and objectives of the organization; the scope of the impact across the organizational structure; the number and relationships of personnel involved; the involvement of external actors such as clients, suppliers, or other stakeholders; and level of emotional response aroused. In resolving conflict, it is clear that there is not a "one size fits all" mechanism available to address the breadth of conflict challenges facing the public health manager. Conflicts can be resolved by a manager through a multitude of tools, including negotiation, counseling, mediation, diplomacy, advocacy, community building, and even prayer. Additionally, beyond the control of the manager, organizations can also pursue conflict resolution through litigation and mediation. Negotiation, a sophisticated technique for conflict resolution, is examined in depth later in this chapter. The following six techniques have excellent application within the environment of the public health manager.

1. *Counseling.* This technique is often utilized in employee relations conflict resolution. A supervisory manager may use counseling in dealing with an issue of a subordinate employee. Counseling sessions involve presentation of the aspects of an issue that the supervisor has determined is creating conflict within an organization. Often, this involves behavioral actions or attitudes on the part of the employee that interfere with the normal activities of the organization. The focus of counseling is to have the employee recognize and accept those aspects of his or her behavior that are creating conflict. The goal is to mutually determine a future course of action that aligns the employee's behavior with the needs of the organization. The personnel manager dealing with a rude receptionist is a conflict example that can often be adequately resolved through counseling.

2. *Mediation.* A conflict between two employees can often be resolved through the technique of mediation. The purpose of mediation is to have the employees mutually agree on a resolution of the conflict. The process to achieve agreement is supervised by a third party acting as a mediator. This person may be the organizational superior of the employees, such as their supervisor or another higher-level actor in the organization, such as a staff member in the HR department. Alternately, it can be a disinterested third party, often from outside the organization. The advantage of using an external third-party mediator is that this person does not generally have a vested interest in the outcome of the mediation, providing a neutral impartiality in the discussions. Additionally, third-party mediators can be specifically chosen for their skills of interpersonal communication, empathy, and knowledge of psychology. The mediation process begins with a set of premises that both parties in conflict must acknowledge for the mediation process to be effective. These premises include:

   - Acknowledgement of conflict between the individuals.
   - Reluctance for the resolution of the conflict to be imposed by a third party.
   - Willingness to work together in a structured manner toward resolution.
   - Acceptance of the presentation of the "other side" of the conflict.
   - Desire to achieve a resolution of the conflict.
   - Agreement to achieve a resolution of the conflict through the guidance of a neutral party.

With acceptance of these premises, the mediation process is then initiated. The process itself will be adapted to the specific conflict and the employees involved, but all mediation processes generally involve these crucial elements in achieving resolution:

- A neutral environment is chosen that does not threaten the participation of either employee.
- The employees are permitted to explain their side of the conflict.
- The mediator referees the discussion to ensure that the presentations are based on individual perspectives and are not attacks on either party.
- The mediator will recap the presentations to facilitate an identification of the issues that can be accepted by all parties to the conflict.
- Discussion will follow that more thoroughly identifies the concerns of each party, and potentially illuminates the goal that each party wishes to achieve.
- The mediator will attempt to frame these competing visions into objective values.
- The mediator will facilitate the identification of options that may lead to achievement of these values.
- The mediator will identify various solutions that incorporate the options presented.
- The employees must then mutually agree on a solution that is acceptable to both of them.
- As a conclusion to the mediation, the solution is typically documented. The documentation is given to all parties to the mediation and also to relevant stakeholders, such as the employees' superior in the organization, and the HR department.

The example of two supervisors competing for staff resources, complaining to the community service clinic manager, is a common conflict situation that is best resolved through mediation. In this example, the manager may not be the appropriate person to perform the mediation. Because both supervisors report to the manager, the ability to maintain impartiality in guiding the mediation is best achieved by utilizing an uninvolved third-party source. This could be the manager of another department of the clinic, the director of the HR department, or an outside mediator.

3. *Diplomacy.* Diplomacy is similar to mediation, in that a third party directs the communication between employees in conflict resolution. The notable difference is that the communication is filtered through the diplomat, who represents to each party the concerns, conflicts, and objectives of the other party in the conflict.

This strategy has the advantage of removing personalities from the resolution of the conflict and allows for dispassionate examination of the causes of the conflict, as well as potential solutions. There is also a time element, in that communication between the two parties takes longer for a diplomat to relay pertinent information than it does through direct communication. This can allow for reflection and reduction of the interpersonal behavioral aspects of a conflict. There are several disadvantages to utilizing diplomacy in conflict resolution. First, the time element can be a disadvantage if the conflict continues to interfere with the achievement of organizational goals until it is resolved. In healthcare organizations such as community service clinics, conflicts that prevent the clinic from effectively serving clients can have health status consequences for the patients and potentially legal consequences for the organization. Second, diplomatic skills are specialized, and it is not common for organizations to routinely employ personnel with that developed skill set. This requires the organization to seek out and engage a diplomat for conflict resolution. The process not only incurs additional expense for the organization, it also compounds the time factor while a diplomat is acquired and then oriented to the organization, the conflict, and the employees involved. Third, many conflicts involve employees who either work in close proximity or are interrelated in the work processes of the organization. It may not be possible for an organization to separate two employees in conflict to allow the diplomatic method to operate effectively.

4. *Advocacy.* This technique is the pursuit of influencing the outcomes of a conflict. It differs from both counseling and diplomacy in that it moves beyond the concerns of the individuals in a conflict situation to the development of an acceptable outcome for the organization. Often, experts are engaged to examine the merits of competing interests, and they present to the organization arguments for the adoption of one side of a conflict situation. It explicitly vests the resolution of the conflict in a superior party to those in conflict, and does not ensure that consensus is reached in resolving the conflict. It has the advantage of broadening the scope of the conflict by bringing additional actors into the conflict situation, which can develop a larger scope of potential solutions to be evaluated. Additionally, the technique can engage more stakeholders in the consequences of the resolution, which can strengthen the final decision by the supervisor or manager. The disad-

vantage to this technique is that it can lead to factionalism and an increase in the conflict without presenting a resolution for the organization. The challenge for the public health manager in utilizing advocacy to resolve conflicts is that it can degenerate to "taking sides" by many employees without leading to a conflict resolution.

5. *Community building.* This method of conflict resolution was developed by psychiatrist M. Scott Peck in his book, *The Different Drum: Community Making and Peace.* Peck defines *community* as having three elements: inclusiveness, commitment, and consensus. Communities go through four stages of development, or building before achieving these elements. In the context of an organization, those stages are:

- *Pseudocommunity*, where members of the organization pretend to have meaningful relationships with each other, but do not acknowledge differences. They behave as if potential conflicts do not exist.
- *Chaos*, where false pretenses have given way to disagreements and emphasis on differences. This is the stage of community building where organizational conflicts from interpersonal relations become manifest.
- *Emptiness*, a process step where individuals abandon their ego and self-interest and become open to the acceptance of a group identity.
- *True community*, where employees come into empathy with each other. At this stage, individuals gain tacit understanding of each other and acknowledge personal differences while building consensus toward organization goals.

Peck's four-stage process is similar to organizational theory models of team development that characterize the stages of development of effective teams as "forming, storming, norming, performing, and transforming." For the public health manager, this technique has limited application in the resolution of a specific conflict concern. It is more appropriate as a general technique that can be used to establish the organization's environment. If community building is actively pursued by management, the climate for conflict is substantially reduced. The use of "morning huddles" by nursing staffs in hospitals serves not only to inform employees of the status of their patients and necessary tasks to be performed during the upcoming shift, it also reinforces the community of care that the organization represents. The use of strategic planning retreats is another venue available to the public health manager to pursue the creation of community within the healthcare organization.

6. *Prayer.* The concept of prayer as a technique for conflict resolution would not intuitively appear to be a tool available to the pubic health manager. The separation of religious and professional behavior is widespread throughout healthcare organizations, with the exception of religious-based institutions such as Catholic hospitals. Nevertheless, prayer in the broadest sense can be used to resolve conflict. The essence of prayer is to focus individuals on something outside of and larger than their own existence and concerns. Elements of prayer do include worship, but they also include requests for assistance and guidance, acknowledgement of personal shortcomings, and provides a method to express thoughts and emotions. Whether termed prayer or "contemplative reflection," this technique allows individuals in a conflict situation to remove ego elements and examine the larger issues involved both in the conflict situation and in its resolution. Public health managers can request a contemplative review by employees in a conflict situation prior to examining issues that require resolution. At its most effective use, such reflection can lead to self-awareness of personal contributions in a conflict and an understanding of the actions, opinions, and concerns of others. At a minimum, the request allows for a "cooling off" period that can dampen or remove emotional responses as the manager seeks to find solutions to the sources of conflict.

NEGOTIATION

The Concept of Negotiation

Negotiation is defined as a deliberative process in which two or more parties enter into discussion for the purpose of achieving an agreement that is advantageous to all participants. It is important to note that there is an expectation of advantage and success on the part of all participants. If someone did not believe that he or she could obtain an advantage in a negotiation, there would be no reason to pursue the process. If you are stopped for speeding, and it is clear that you have no opportunity to convince the officer of either the facts of your action or its merits, there is no advantage to be obtained from negotiating. But most people believe that there may be the chance that they can convince an officer to not write up a speeding ticket, or perhaps only issue a warning. Hence, they begin a conversation, which is a negotiation. Similarly in health care, certain actions are not amenable to negotiation. The requirement of proper licensure for healthcare providers is not negotiable with state or federal authorities that are responsible for ensuring the safety of health services patients. But the final report and recommendations of an accrediting body such as the Joint Commission on Accreditation of Healthcare Organizations (JCAHO) can potentially be negotiated if the public health manager can successfully argue for evidence of demonstrable progress in meeting accreditation standards. And something as routine as hiring a lab technician is, in fact, a negotiation. How much you are willing to pay in wages and benefits is a point of discussion in the hiring process. Often, an organization has strict pay scales that do not allow for flexibility in compensation, but the creative public health manager may determine that the potential employee would accept the position if her scheduled working hours can be shifted slightly to accommodate child care needs. Thus, negotiation is present even in the most structured aspects of an organization.

Successful negotiation requires planning, strategy, and execution. All three elements are critical to the negotiation process, but none are beyond the ability of the public health manager willing to commit time and effort to the process. The following sections discuss these elements in detail.

Negotiation Planning—Developing Preferences and Alternatives

Successful negotiation is not something that just "happens," either through the persuasive personality of a negotiator or the fortuitousness of superior elements available to the negotiator. Success begins with *planning*, and in negotiation the first component of the planning process is to determine if it is appropriate to enter into a negotiation. As discussed in the samples provided earlier, no one is *required* to negotiate, and if no advantage can be obtained, then the resources employed in negotiations are best utilized elsewhere. The manager who believes there is a reason to negotiate has assumed that there is an advantage (profit) to be gained from the negotiation. But for a negotiation to occur, there are several conditions to be met. Johnson (1993) has identified these as:

- The active involvement of at least two parties.
- An understanding by involved parties of the negotiation as a method to reach a goal.
- The willingness of involved parties to develop and exchange proposals to obtain a settlement.
- An understanding by each party that he or she expects to profit from the exchange.

Once a determination has been made that an environment for negotiation exists, the manager needs to work through a series of pre-negotiation steps. These steps will allow the manager to determine the framework though which the negotiation process will proceed. These steps include:

- Identifying negotiation opportunities.
- Determining interests.
- Determining alternatives.
- Analyzing relevant information.
- Assessing strengths and weaknesses.
- Choosing negotiation strategies and communication styles.
- Considering mechanisms to achieve win–win outcomes.

Identification of negotiation opportunities is often the most neglected aspect of the pre-negotiation process. Managers routinely assume that terms, conditions, and prices are fixed beyond the ability of the manager to moderate. But as previously discussed, many items confronting the public health manager are opportunities for negotiation. The director of a county health department may go to a cell phone kiosk and bargain for additional free minutes in exchange for renewing a cellular telephone contract. But that same director may not make the connection that the telephone service for the entire health department is also negotiable.

The pertinent question in planning shifts from whether an item *is* negotiable to whether it is *in the interest* of the organization to engage in negotiation. For the pubic health manager, a simple rule of thumb states that "if an organization can be improved by the increase of a resource," that resource should be considered a target for negotiation. Note that the concept of *increase* here means more than the abundance of positive items for the organization, such as more revenue from a client services contract, more services from a photocopier lease agreement, or more benefits within the premium structure of a health insurance contract. It also denotes the reduction of constraints to the organization, such as lengthening a specific time period for reporting to outside agencies, relief from onerous regulations that divert staff and resources from the organization's mission, or the ability to shift staff members to different work sites or responsibilities without being required by a union to add additional employees.

Once an appropriate negotiation opportunity has been identified, the next step for the public health manager is to identify interests. This involves understanding not only the tangible items of interest, such as money and rules, but also the intangible items of interest such as respect, self-image, and motivation. These tangible and intangible interests influence the manager's determination of what he or she wants from an opportunity, and also allow the manager to rank the importance of those items. For example, it may be that a medical

clinic manager wants a 10% overall increase in payments from an insurance company for the services provided by the clinic, but it may also be the case that the manager would like an easier approval process to provide diagnostic procedures to the insured. Pre-negotiation in this example would involve specifying all of the potential results that can be achieved through the negotiation process and then specifying the preferred rank order of the listed items. One item that should always be included and ranked is the creation (or continuance) of a relationship with the other party in the negotiation. Making a determination of the importance of the relationship has significant consequences in negotiation strategy, as we will see later. In addition to understanding your interests in the negotiation, it is also important to understand the interests and rankings of the other party. The simple exercise of "putting yourself in their shoes" may provide insight into what the other party values and can determine the strategy process that the manager pursues.

A prioritized ranking of interests leads to the development of alternatives in the negotiation process. Alternatives have two meanings in this context—one as options in the negotiation process and the other as the difference between an agreement and the best position in the absence of an agreement. *Options* are opportunities to change the nature of the environment being negotiated so that both parties can profit from the negotiation. In referring to the medical fee schedule example, the medical group's interest in obtaining a 10% increase in fee reimbursement is in opposition to the interest of an insurance company holding down increases in costs that must be recaptured through higher insurance premiums. But an option might be that the medical practice requests an increase only in the payments it receives for primary care services and agrees to increase its capacity to provide those services. Both parties to the negotiation have an opportunity for gain: the medical practice can increase its revenue for some services and expand its business, while the insurance company can market the availability of more primary care services to its enrollees, and potentially increase the number of people choosing the company for health insurance coverage, thus increasing its revenue to cover the additional costs. Strategically, the use of options that expand the negotiation sphere creates opportunities for win–win situations. The concept is to avoid zero-sum strategies, where one party wins only at the expense of the other party.

The other concept of alternative is often referred to as the "best alternative to a negotiated agreement" or BATNA. It is not always the case that the best outcome can be achieved through negotiation. As previously discussed, the purpose of negotiation is to satisfy defined interests, and it may be the case that interests are better served through the best alternative to a negotiated agreement. The BATNA represents the best method to achieve the defined interests without requiring the other party's agreement. Fisher and Ury (1991) and Ury (1991) developed the BATNA model in *Getting to Yes*. Their framework suggests that having a BATNA creates leverage and is the key to negotiating power. The stronger the BATNA, the more power the party has in negotiations. The concept is not a "bottom line" of the minimum that one party would accept in a negotiation. Instead, it is the alternative action of moving away from a negotiation.

For example, assume a public health manager is attempting to obtain a grant to provide screening services to an underserved inner-city population. In response to his inquiry, the funding agency has suggested making available a grant of $1,000,000 to provide a comprehensive set of services, beyond the current capacity of the community clinic. The manager reviews the requirements and estimates that the cost to the agency to provide these additional services would be greater than the expected grant. A bottom-line approach would be an insistence by the manager that the services could not be provided for less than $1,200,000. But a BATNA approach would be to examine what would happen if the grant was not accepted. Could limited funding be acquired from a competing agency to initiate a pilot program of the services? Could the agency curtail certain services it is currently providing to accommodate new services? The advantage of working from a BATNA is that it allows the flexibility to explore options that may not be apparent in the dichotomous decision matrix suggest in the bottom-line stance. The problem with a bottom-line approach is that although it may protect the public health manager from accepting a bad settlement, it prevents the manager from creating and accepting a solution that is preferable to the alternative outside of the negotiation. The critical steps in the BATNA strategy are:

1. *Identify the BATNA.* In other words, what alternatives will exist if the manager walks away from the negotiation? There are three elements to this process:

   - Creating a list of what will be done if an agreement is not reached.
   - Working through the list to develop these ideas into obtainable alternatives.
   - Making a tentative selection of the one alternative that is the best.

2. *Increase the strength of the chosen alternative.* The degree to which this choice outside the negotiation can be objectively specified in terms of costs and outcomes determines how strong it becomes as an alternative position to the offers made in the negotiation.

3. *Determine if there is a need to negotiate.* In many instances, the alternative may be better than what could be obtained through negotiation, especially when the costs to negotiate are included in the evaluation.

4. *Examine the potential BATNA of the other side.* This exercise provides insight into the level of agreement that must be overcome to exceed the BATNA of the other party. The more the manager knows about the alternatives available to the other party, the better prepared the manager can be for negotiation. It will also give an indication of the relative strength or weakness of the other party's BATNA. This information is useful in assessing the expectations the other party will set in negotiation.

In analyzing the relevant information, the public health manager must look beyond the negotiation specifics to the larger context for all parties involved, not just those in the actual negotiation. It is here that stakeholder analysis, historic or corporate precedent, cultural concerns, and value and belief systems must be taken into consideration. In the BATNA example previously discussed, the public health manager reviewed a revenue gap between the agency funding that was available and the anticipated costs of implementing a comprehensive set of services. The analysis of relevant information would also include community expectations that the clinic would provide those services. A stakeholder analysis of staff, board members, community organizers, political figures, and other healthcare institution representatives would also be conducted to evaluate the impact on the clinic of a decision to proceed or not proceed with the new service program. Cultural expectations would provide important information about the ability of the clinic to successfully implement the program. And finally, knowledge of the success of similar programs, the history of the clinic's relationship with the funding agency, and the clinic's own experience in establishing new programs would all be relevant information to be analyzed in preparation for negotiations.

An analysis of the strengths and weaknesses of the other party, as well as the manager's own position, is required to place the negotiation within the bargaining zone. If expectations of either party exceed the potential to reach agreement, this weakness needs to be evaluated in the context of the BATNA. A SWOT analysis from the perspective of both parties will reveal options that can be exploited in the negotiation process. A SWOT analysis examines the *strengths* and *weaknesses* inside an organization, as well as the *opportunities* and *threats* outside the organization. For example, if the public health manager analyzes the environment of the funding agency and determines that the agency will be evaluated on the breadth and depth of its grants within the current fiscal year, that constraint becomes a weakness to the funding agency, but it simultaneously represents an opportunity to the community service clinic. A previously conducted pilot program of similar services can represent a strength for the community service clinic and an opportunity for the funding agency.

Negotiation Strategy—Emphasis on Relationships Versus Issues

Choosing negotiation strategies and communication styles is crucial to an effective negotiation process. Johnson (1993) outlines four major strategies that are typically utilized in successful negotiation: soft bargaining, hard bargaining, tit-for-tat bargaining, and principled bargaining. The choice of negotiation strategy involves both the preference of the negotiator and the appropriateness of the situation. The *soft approach* is based on the development of relationships during the negotiation process as opposed to the emphasis on issues or points of conflict. This approach may be appropriate in negotiations that do not have significant consequences for the parties involved. In choosing a photocopier lease from a supplier that represents several brands, the soft approach may allow both parties to reach an advantageous solution without risking the larger stake of a continuing relationship.

Minimizing the importance of the relationships for the importance of the issue is the basis for the *hard approach*. Here, the negotiator can take advantage of strength in the face of weakness to impose an agreement, and the approach is well suited for short-term relationships, or where there are multiple alternative negotiations available. The negotiation of a contract for office supplies can be a "take it or leave it" offer from the public health manager if there are multiple sources of office supplies competing for the health agency's business.

The *tit-for-tat approach* works from a sense of fairness. Giving an incremental concession to the other party in exchange for a similar concession is a strategy that allows both sides to build a trust relationship during the course of the negotiation. It is particularly useful in situations where there have been prior relationship difficulties between the parties or when both parties are new to the negotiation and are seeking a long-term relationship beyond the current negotiation.

Principled bargaining involves establishing a method that respects parties in the relationship and focuses on the broad interests of both parties. Its focus is to broaden the scope of the negotiation and develop agreements that are characterized as win–win. It is particularly applicable when there is an imbalance of power between the negotiating parties, either from the strength of the respective positions, or the strength of the personalities engaged in negotiation. Johnson's evaluation of the characteristics, strengths, and weaknesses of each strategy is summarized in the following sections.

The Strategy of Soft Bargaining

Characteristics of the negotiator:

- Agreeability, flexibility, avoidance of conflict and unpleasant exchanges.
- They adopt a conciliatory attitude, and expect reciprocity in negotiations. Their tools revolve around appeals to personalities and relationships and include using guilt, sympathy, and implied threats.
- Their arguments appeal to cooperation, agreement, and team play.

Advantages of the soft bargaining strategy:

- Powerful attraction for people searching for a comfortable relationship. Negotiators can gain an advantage with these people, especially in creating a sense of obligation to reciprocate in bargaining.
- Creation of a sense of mutual dependence, with the potential of mutual self-sacrifice to create a mutual benefit.
- Evidence indicates that soft bargaining can be more successful in creating agreement when negotiations have reached a deadlock. A softer approach can lead to more flexibility in the search for solutions.
- Soft bargaining can be an effective response to strong personalities, in that deference can create a more approachable response from "high maintenance" negotiators.

Disadvantages of the soft bargaining strategy:

- Soft bargaining may not be effective when the negotiator is functioning as a representative of others. The soft approach may cost the representative credibility with client parties, who typically expect their interests to be handled with strong advocacy.
- It may not be effective against a hard bargaining strategy by the other party in the negotiation. Hard bargainers can take advantage of the concessionary tactics of the soft bargainer without moving toward consensus.
- Soft bargaining can lead to unnecessary concessions to create a relationship in the negotiation. Opposing parties can take advantage of this and increase their demands.
- Sustaining credibility over time can be difficult, in that negotiators might conclude that a relationship was created simply for the soft bargainer to be exploited for nonreciprocal gain.

The Strategy of Hard Bargaining

Characteristics of the negotiator:

- Toughness, rigidity, adversarial approach employing techniques of intimidation and attempts of forceful coercion.
- They use the technique both as a style and as a tactic to forgo making concessions or incremental retreats.
- They use the force of their personalities, either overtly or through silent intransigence to gain advantage in negotiation.
- They exchange points in negotiation on predefined terms and view the negotiation as a contest to maximize only their own gain.

Advantages of the hard bargaining strategy:

- The straightforward style without subtle or hidden agendas provides strength to the hard bargainer that gives power in the negotiation process.
- Research indicates that a hard bargaining style produces results when the negotiator is viewed as credible. Success in achieving concessions through this style is positively related to negotiators who are perceived as possessing attractiveness and high esteem.
- Hard bargaining negotiation can preclude the opposing party from developing potential alternatives. Continual forcefulness in negotiation can lead to premature concession from opposing parties, who evaluate the psychological cost of continued negotiation beyond the potential advantages to be gain from continued discussion.

Disadvantages of the hard bargaining strategy:

- Hard bargaining may result in the loss of relationships. This aggressive style has interpersonal consequences that can damage the level of interaction necessary to conduct successful negotiations as a continuing activity. It may lead to an unwillingness to engage in future negotiations.
- Hard bargaining may be met with hard bargaining from other negotiators willing to be even more aggressive in pursuit of the strategy.
- It can lead to a loss of credibility. Hard bargaining often utilizes overt or implied threats. Unwillingness to properly carry through appropriate threat postures can reduce the credibility, and the effectiveness, of the negotiator.
- A common response to hard bargainers is avoidance. Opposing negotiators may choose attempt to negotiate with another party or choose to forgo negotiation completely.
- Hard bargaining can lead to missed opportunities for easy gain. An inflexible approach can preclude accepting a lesser offer that could still represent a profit for the negotiator.

The Strategy of Tit-for-Tat Bargaining

Characteristics of the negotiator:

- Reciprocity, incremental focus, second mover, appeals to rationality and equitable exchange.
- They adopt a response tactic that matches the initial move by an opposing negotiator. Positive first moves are met with positive responses, and likewise with negative moves.
- They are attempting to provide a scenario where reward is met with reward, punishment is met with punishment, and where they have the ability to control these exchanges.

Advantages of the tit-for-tat bargaining strategy:

- The strategy creates a sense of predictability, which allows parties to clearly understand and respond with a certainty of the reactions to their responses.
- Tit-for-tat may be effective in shaping behavior in a Skinnerian methodology of positive and negative reinforcement.
- It may remove the effect of personality in the opponent's bargaining style. Neither the soft appeal to mutual concern nor the hard appeal of threats and intimidation are effective in shaping the responses from a tit-for-tat negotiator.

Disadvantages of the tit-for-tat bargaining strategy:

- In being a responsive second mover, the negotiator forgoes control of initial positions in a negotiation.
- The strategy precludes the negotiation of a large advantage, or domination, by the negotiator. Equitable agreements are the logical outcome of this bargaining style.
- Progress toward mutual gain may not be achievable if the opposing negotiator is hostile toward the tit-for-tat approach or pursues a stringent hard bargaining position of winning at any cost.
- Determining the appropriate level of responsive reward or punishment is difficult, with the result that tactical maneuvers may not result in the desired level of response.

- The flow of tit-for-tat negotiation may lead to a deferral of pursing the desired advantages in a timely or cost-effective framework.

The Strategy of Principled Bargaining

Characteristics of the negotiator:

- Focuses on problems rather than people, focuses on interests not positions, seeks options for mutual gain, and utilizes objective standards.
- Agreeability, flexibility, avoidance of conflict and unpleasant exchanges.
- They adopt a conciliatory attitude and expect reciprocity in negotiations.
- Their tools revolve around appeals to personalities and relationships and include using guilt, sympathy, and implied threats. Their arguments appeal to cooperation, agreement, and team play.

Advantages of the principled bargaining strategy:

- Powerful attraction for people searching for a comfortable relationship. Negotiators can gain an advantage with these people, especially in creating a sense of obligation to reciprocate in bargaining.
- Creation of a sense of mutual dependence, with the potential of mutual self-sacrifice to create a mutual benefit.
- Evidence indicates that soft bargaining can be more successful in creating agreement when negotiations have reached a deadlock. A softer approach can lead to more flexibility in the search for solutions.
- Soft bargaining can be an effective response to strong personalities, in that deference can create a more approachable response from "high maintenance" negotiators.

Disadvantages of principled bargaining strategy:

- Soft bargaining may not be effective when the negotiator is functioning as a representative of others. The soft approach may cost the representative credibility with client parties, who typically expect their interests to be handled with strong advocacy.
- It may not be effective against a hard bargaining strategy by the other party in the negotiation. Hard bargainers can take advantage of concessionary tactics of the soft bargainer, without moving toward consensus.
- Soft bargaining can lead to unnecessary concessions to create a relationship in the negotiation. Opposing parties can take advantage of this and increase their demands.

- Sustaining credibility over time can be difficult, in that negotiators might conclude that a relationship was created simply for the soft bargainer to be exploited for nonreciprocal gain.

Negotiation Execution—Tactics

Choosing the bargaining strategy to be employed in a negotiation, after negotiation planning, is the second aspect of the process. The third aspect is the use of negotiation tactics within the strategic framework. Fisher and Ury (1991) and Ury (1991) delineate a series of "tricky tactics" used by negotiators that they note can be divided into three categories: deliberate deception, psychological warfare, and positional pressure. In understanding these tactics and how they are employed, the public healthcare manager can adapt them to his or her advantage in the negotiation process.

Deliberate deception is the conscious effort to present information or factual statements that do not present a true picture of the environment of the negotiation. While ethical considerations affect the use of deception as a business practice, judicial employment of deception can lead an opponent to agreement with your position in a negotiation. Fisher and Ury note three types of deception: the presentation of false statements, the appeal of ambiguous authority, and withholding pertinent information. Presenting false statements can be used to paint a picture that the opponent in a negotiation might desire. For example, in asking for increased fees for specific surgical procedures, a medical practice administrator might state to an insurance company that "We really don't do many of these procedures, but when we do, we need to be compensated much more than we are at this time. It's the only way we can attract the best-trained surgeons to join our practice." The facts may be that the practice does a substantial number of the procedures, but it is the responsibility of the opposing negotiator to make that determination. This tactic also suggests that each negotiator should be skeptical of any factual claims made in a negotiation. Separating opinions of negotiators from information presented suggests that "trust but verify" is the core component of this negotiation tactic.

Deception also involves implying that the negotiator possesses full authority to complete the negotiation. Working through a negotiation as if you can finalize an agreement but withholding final approval to the acceptance of a superior allows for maneuvering after an opponent's best position has been revealed. The classic example of this involves the back-and-forth discussion with an automotive salesperson. Numbers are recorded on a sales document that appears to represent a completed negotiation, but inevitably the salesperson has to "run this by my manager." This tactic reserves the ability for the negotiator to press for additional advantage. When confronted with this tactic, the best response is to demand reciprocity in opening previously agreed points in a negotiation to reconsideration by both parties.

Similar to deception is the tactic of less than full disclosure. Negotiation does not require the disclosure of all facts, especially if doing so would put the negotiator at a disadvantage. In the example presented earlier regarding negotiation for surgical procedure fees, both parties could, and should, verify the number of procedures currently being performed. But the medical practice administrator is under no obligation to disclose during negotiation that the group has hired a new surgeon who specializes in those procedures, which will increase the volume above current levels after the negotiations are completed.

Various *psychological tactics* can also be used to advantage by the negotiator. The imposition of stress on opposing negotiators can be useful in moving them to accept positions to your advantage. The tactics of inducing stress include manipulating the physical environment of the negotiation arena, insisting that negotiations take place in a space the negotiator controls instead of a neutral location, and bringing a superior number of participants into the negotiations as a show of force. The use of these tactics can distract a negotiator from focusing on negotiating points to focusing on personal comfort concerns (physical, psychological, or social) that results in agreements or concessions not in that negotiator's best interests. When confronted with these tactics, the best response may to be to call a "time out" from negotiations to reestablish a comfort zone (in every sense) acceptable to you prior to engaging in meaningful discussions.

Another psychological tactic is the "ad hominem," or personal attack. This tactic has many forms and variations, but its essential trait is to move the discussion from the issues to some aspect of the opposing negotiator. Commenting on the personal appearance of the negotiator, questioning the knowledge or expertise of the negotiator, or even ignoring the presence of the negotiator to deal with trivial matters all give the impression that the opposing negotiator is not an equal in the discussions. This puts the opposing negotiator in the position of having to first establish the validity of being a party to the negotiation prior to engaging in exchanges of the points of contention. This tactic can be useful in that the responding negotiator will often concede points in the negotiation process to establish his or her legitimacy as a participant in the discussions. In negotiating funding for a new public health agency service, the public health manager might comment on the larger health policy issues driving changes in service delivery. With an opposing negotiator focused on budgetary and accounting policies (which is often the situation), the public

health manager can gain a superior negotiating position. This discussion can highlight the potential knowledge disadvantage of the financially based negotiator. The public health manager can suggest that agreeing to certain funding points is not only appropriate for the goals of the program, but also gives the opposing negotiator an opportunity to be perceived as aware of larger concerns, thus enhancing the negotiator's reputation in the public health service community.

The final psychological tactic is the "good guy–bad guy" routine. A well-established method, this tactic requires two participants on one side of the negotiation, with the "bad guy" primarily employing the hard bargaining strategy previously described. After the presentation of uncompromising points from this negotiator, the second participant, or the "good guy," utilizes the soft bargaining strategy to suggest a concession that potentially would be accepted by the hard bargainer. This tactic is employed to make the opposing negotiator agree to this point, which has been made to appear reasonable by contrast to the initial position. Resisting this tactic requires a consistent response to both negotiators, putting forward the same response in reply to the suggestion of the "good guy" that would be offered to the negotiating partner.

Fisher and Ury conclude their examination of negotiation tactics by delineating *positional pressure tactics*, which involve structuring the negotiation arena in such a manner that the ability to concede points is limited to the opponent in the negotiation. The most common positional tactic is the refusal to negotiate. A key component of the hard bargaining strategy, this tactic may be employed to make the opponent concede points before entering into a tit-for-tat bargaining strategy. The tactic is usually countered by confronting the refusal to negotiate, using third-party communication for negotiations, or moving to a principled bargaining strategy.

Setting outlier demands or conditions is another positional tactic that lowers expectations and can move negotiations into a mutually beneficial zone of discussion. In the example of the medical practice administrator negotiating for higher surgical procedure reimbursements, an initial insistence on substantial increases (e.g., double the rate of inflation) may be a mechanism to move discussion into a pricing structure that can meet the needs of the practice and work within the budget of the insurance company. The drawback to this tactic is that making a demand that is perceived as too extreme can undermine the credibility of the negotiator. A countertactic to outlier demands would be to point out the inappropriateness of the position through the demonstration of similar extreme demands. Alternately, the tactic can be countered by a stated withdrawal from negotiations until suggestions within a zone of mutual interest are presented.

Continuing to increase demands on certain points in response to agreement on other points is also a positional pressure tactic that can be employed. This tactic includes reopening previously agreed positions. By continually rearranging the points of agreement, the negotiator may move the total zone of acceptance to his or her advantage. The counter to this tactic involves bargaining from principles and insisting that agreements on points cannot be disavowed to bargain on open items in a negotiation. Consider the situation of a public health manager who is negotiating price, delivery, and payment terms of vaccines to be used in a local clinic. Unit price might be agreed upon early in the discussion, but the manager may insist that the price be reduced upon completion of the payment schedule discussion. The supplier is then faced with either renegotiating the price or offering more attractive terms of payment, or both. But this tactic can be ineffective if the manager does not have an alternative source of the vaccine.

The lock-in is a positional pressure tactic that is the negotiation equivalent of "playing chicken." The negotiator establishes what is presented as an intractable position and, in essence, dares the opposing negotiator to change toward that position or risk the collapse of the entire negotiation. This is an extreme tactic, and it again places the negotiator into a potential situation of loss of credibility if he or she is forced to move from the locked-in position. The tactic has the advantage of clearly establishing the commitment of the negotiator to a position, but it limits the availability of alternative positions to which the negotiator can move. It can be countered by pointing out that the lock-in position focuses on the status of the negotiator staking the claim, and not on the issue at hand to be resolved.

The use of delay can be a successful positional pressure tactic. All negotiations have an element of time, and the negotiator who can use the pressure of time has a distinct advantage in the negotiation. Managers should recognize that salespeople are often evaluated on performance measures that are compiled on a monthly or quarterly basis. If a public health manager is considering the purchase of an electronic health record, delaying conclusion of the negotiation until the end of the supplier's accounting period can result in additions to service packages or reductions in fees to complete the sale. The negotiator needs to recognize the two-sided aspect of using delay as a tactic. If a time period critical to the opposing negotiator passes, the opposing negotiator may be uninterested or unable to effectively continue in the negotiation.

Finally, the negotiator can establish a "take-it-or-leave-it" position. This is often a tactic of finality, where the negotiator has concluded that the stated position is marginally better than a previously determined BATNA. If the opposing party is un-

willing to accept the point, then the negotiator is prepared to terminate the discussions and move to the best alternative to a negotiated agreement. This tactic also implies that there is no longer an agreement zone where further negotiation is possible, and in many situations this can be the opening position. Retail sales are typically take-or-leave situations, without a zone for negotiation. As a response to this tactic, a negotiator can continue to proceed as if the position was not stated by introducing alternative solutions. Alternately, this tactic can be countered by pointing out that "leave it" may leave both parties worse off than what could be established through further negotiations.

CONCLUSION

The public health manager will face situations of both conflict and negotiation in the pursuit of organizational goals. In developing an appropriate response, the primary consideration is that the manager work from the position of determining what course of action is best suited to advance the mission of the organization. That analysis will guide the subsequent decision processes and actions that have been described in processing conflict and negotiating on behalf of the organization. Once a course of action has been chosen, it remains for the public health manager to choose to act or to allow the situation to proceed without direction. And in certain instances, this latter choice may be the most appropriate for the organization.

A concluding consideration is the cost of conflict resolution and negotiation. The manager faces resource constraints involving financial limitations; the diversion of personnel, including themselves and those affected in a conflict or a negotiation; and the use of precious time in pursuing the course of action. All of these represent opportunity costs to the manager. Other options cannot be chosen, other alternatives cannot be pursued with the resources that the manager brings to the negotiation or resolution action. The public health manager must weigh the value of active participation in these actions against the other activities that could be undertaken to achieve organizational goals. And once involved in a negotiation process, resources will continue to be used. If a negotiation continues without a timely resolution that meets the established needs of the organization, a manager must decide whether to continue to commit the organization's resources to obtain the desired ends. The criticality of the BATNA analysis is that it provides a "cut-off" point for the manager to evaluate the return on committing additional resources to the process.

A core component of leadership for management is the prudent utilization of an organization's resources in pursuit of its mission. Thus, the manager must consider not only the ends to be achieved, but also the degree to which the organization's resources should be used to achieve these ends. Conflict resolution and negotiation are vital tools to be mastered by the public healthcare manager. They can only be mastered through experience gained by practice. Conflict resolution is never easy and is often uncomfortable due to the inherent friction of interpersonal activities. Negotiation is a skill that requires different approaches for different situations and can often be bluntly applied where a delicate touch would be more effective, or vice versa. But successful leadership in public health management requires both prudent discretion in the utilization of these tools and experienced skill in their application.

CLOSING THOUGHTS AND FURTHER READINGS

The basic structure of both conflict resolution and negotiation require the public health manager to create a situation in which both parties conclude an interaction with a sense of positive gain. This is the concept of creating a win–win situation. The public health manager will seek to create win–win situations, where the winners are not only the individuals involved, but the institutions they represent as well as significant stakeholders in the broader industry sphere. Managers who look for leadership opportunities will attempt to develop negotiation strategies and conflict resolution approaches to create solutions that are larger than the simple sum of their conclusions.

The literature in this regard is extensive, and there are several texts that are regularly cited for their insight in developing these tools. Howard Raffia's *The Art and Science of Negotiation* presents a series of essays that explore negotiation from a qualitative basis through case studies and a quantitative basis of mathematical modeling to explore negotiation strategies and responses. *Win–Win Negotiating: Turning Conflict into Agreement*, by Fred Jandt, presents scenarios of negotiation and conflict resolution from real-world situations, such as labor negotiators, diplomats, and corporate managers. And finally, the classic of creating both the win–win concept of negotiation and the BATNA concept is Roger Fisher and William Ury's *Getting to Yes: Negotiating Agreement Without Giving In*. This short text explores many of the concepts presented here and provides a variety of real-world examples that illustrate the universal application of their principles.

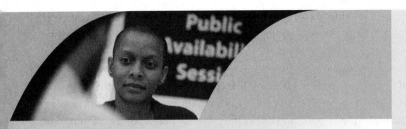

Discussion Questions

1. One issue facing managers is the conflict between "corporate culture" and "social culture." The norms of behavior, communication, dress, and even personal appearance can vary widely between these two frameworks. In healthcare organizations, certain standards of presentation are required due to health concerns (such as policies regarding the use of artificial nails in patient care occupations). However, the manager must also instill organizational values in new employees. Consider the example of an employee with facial piercings. If you are the administrator of a hospice facility, how would you approach discussing with your employee the potential that this may be disruptive to the care processes of the organization? What techniques might be best suited to resolving the differences between freedom of personal expression and the need for patient-focused care in all dimensions (clinical, social, and psychological)?

2. The application of specific mediation techniques must be tempered by not only the specific conflict to be resolved, but also the characteristics of the employees involved. These characteristics include the personal attributes, work values, and social skills of the employees involved and also their status within the organization (work peers, superior versus subordinate, etc.). Consider the situation where an employee comes to you with a lengthy, pointed complaint that a co-worker is not "pulling his weight" in accomplishing the required tasks in a work group. What elements should be considered in creating mediation between these two employees if they are co-workers? What if one employee is the supervisor of the other employee? Is your approach to mediation different based on who (supervisor or subordinate) brings the complaint to your attention?

3. Community building can be particularly effective as a prophylactic mechanism to reduce future conflict in an organization. Although managers may derisively characterize this activity as nothing more than "group hugs," it does create pathways to reinforce the mission and values of an organization. If you are the manager of a community health center in a high-need urban community, how could you use community building as a way to combat the inevitable sense of futility and burn-out faced by employees in that environment? What specific activities would you develop to maintain the "community" among workers in a community health center?

4. As suggested by the discussion on conducting a SWOT analysis of both parties to a negotiation, much can be learned through consideration of the position of the opposing side of a negotiation. "Putting yourself in their shoes" is an exercise that can yield valuable insight in preparing for a negotiation. Consider the example of a funding agency request for new services. Using a BATNA framework, what might be the possible alternatives available to the funding agency outside of the negotiation? What should the managers of the agency do to increase the strength of these options? Does successful negotiation always require knowledge of BATNA options in advance of actual discussion? Are negotiation options limited if a BATNA strategy is not identified in advance? If so, how?

5. The choice of negotiation strategy will be driven by various considerations, including the importance placed on the negotiation by the organization, the economic value of the outcome, the participants involved, the time frame of the negotiation, and the alternatives to negotiation that are available. Given these dimensions of assessing the negotiation process, discuss which strategy would be most appropriate in the following situations, and why.
   - The community health center needs to expand its physical space to provide additional services and is in discussion with the building owner to lease the floor above the center.
   - An invoice is received at a health clinic that lists prices for supplies approximately 15% above what

had been discussed over the telephone when placing the order.

- A marketing company is presenting a proposal to "brand" a medical center with new logos, websites, and promotional material during a two-year campaign.
- A medical internship training program is facing possible probationary status based on the survey findings of an accreditation agency.

6. Negotiation tactics are also dependent on conditions of organizational values, economic expectations, characteristics of the participants, time frames, and negotiation alternatives. In considering the example of a community health center negotiating for additional space for new services, describe which, if any, psychological tactics would be appropriate to employ during the negotiation. Is the tactic aligned with a particular negotiation strategy, or could it be employed with equal effectiveness with any of the negotiation strategies presented? How much does the success of a particular tactic of deception, psychology, or positional pressure depend on the personality of the negotiator? Can these tactics be utilized by any trained person, or are they dependent on the "style" of the individual negotiator?

REFERENCES

Fisher R, Ury W. *Getting to Yes: Negotiating Agreement Without Giving In.* 2nd ed. New York: Penguin Books; 1991:200.

Jandt FE. *Win-Win Negotiating: Turning Conflict into Agreement.* New York: Wiley; 1985:300.

Johnson RA. *Negotiation Basics: Concepts, Skills, and Exercises.* Newbury Park, CA: Sage Publications; 1993:166.

Peck S. *The Different Drum: Community-Making and Peace.* New York: Simon & Schuster; 1987.

Raiffa H. *The Art and Science of Negotiation.* Cambridge, MA: Belknap Press of Harvard University Press; 1982:373.

Ury W. *Getting Past No: Negotiating with Difficult People.* New York: Bantam Books; 1991:161.

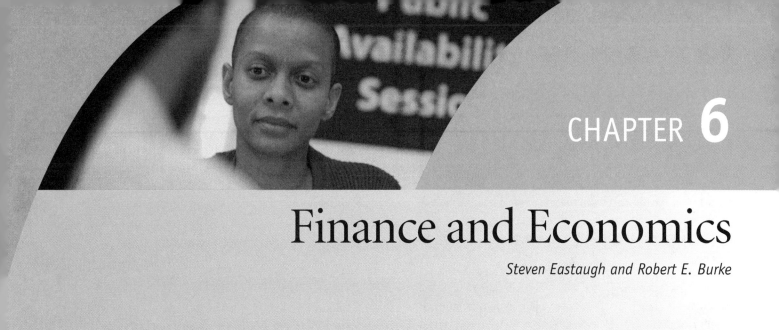

Finance and Economics

Steven Eastaugh and Robert E. Burke

CHAPTER **6**

INTRODUCTION

As a student in public health management, you may be asking the question, "Why is there a chapter on finance and economics?" The answer is quite simple. Without an understanding of the general principles of finance and economics, you will not be an effective manager able to make the decisions and tough choices between and among scarce resources on the day-to-day basics that are required to ensure the successful operation of your public health program. The goal of this chapter is to introduce basic concepts of finance and health economics as applied to American public health. Once you have mastered the basic concepts, the chapter aims to encourage you to delve deeper with additional study of public finance, public health finance, and health economics.

In American culture, expressions such as "Show me the money" and "Follow the money" have entered our everyday language. Without knowledge of how money (finance and economics) operates, it does not matter how noble a health or social program may be; it is doomed to fail. The purpose of this chapter is to provide a framework and a basic understanding of how money moves in and out of public health and to address the specific concerns of the public health manager.

As stated in Chapter 5, one of the roles of the public health manager is to control the assets that are needed to fund public health programs. Public health funding does not just simply appear by the good fortune of some agency. Public health funding is from many sources. A primary function of this chapter is for the public health manager to learn these about these sources—how funding is obtained, planned for, and safe-guarded. The authors agree that to be an effective manager, the manager needs to understand a few principles of finance and economics. These principles come from a long history of research and application. Thus, the next step for the future successful manager is to be able to understand and apply some finance and economic principles.

LEARNING OBJECTIVES

After reading this chapter, the reader will be able to:

1. Describe how public health programs in the Unites States receive funding.
2. Discuss how the principles of finance impact public health management.
3. Describe how principles of economics apply to public health management.

BASICS OF HEALTHCARE FINANCE

The section begins with a brief history on how public health programs are paid for in the United States. The chapter then presents the issues of public health finance, followed by a presentation of how state and federal government agencies financially support public health. After the examples of public health finance are presented, the chapter concludes with a discussion of how healthcare economics are applied to public health.

Other chapters explain management theory and concepts. The sources for public health programs are presented. This chapter describes how those functions are related to the financing and economics of public health management.

There are two major concerns of finance: (1) how money is allocated or sent to an organization so that it can perform its function or do its stated and approved work, and (2) how to determine the different sources of funding. Money to run a public health enterprise does not simply appear. In the most basic terms, the money to run the enterprise comes from both public agencies, including local, state, and federal governments, and from private sources, such as donations from individuals and philanthropic organizations. In the United States, the local, state, and federal governments—by means of an elaborate set of formulas—determine the allocation of dollars to meet the public health needs of an area or region. Not all regions or public health enterprises receive the same amount of funding. The different rationales for these differences are discussed later in this chapter.

FINANCING HEALTH CARE AND RESOURCE ALLOCATION

In the United States, the public health enterprise has its own history. The different financing arrangements reflect this history. The first question policy makers need to ask is, How much of the available money should and could be allocated to public health tasks? In a capitalistic society, the question could be framed as, How much investment needs to be made by both public and private sectors to maintain and grow the economy? For a capitalistic society to thrive and grow, assets need to be set aside to ensure we have a healthy workforce. In addition to those currently working, the pipeline of future workers needs to be healthy. When the business enterprise is growing more quickly than the number of current workers and the pipeline of future workers cannot deliver new workers fast enough to meet the need, then one solution is to import workers from foreign countries who are healthy and will not bring disease or contaminate the existing and current workforce. Over the years, the health of these employees was a task that became the purview of public health.

Regardless of who benefits from the local and state public health offices, just how is the public health enterprise funded? Elected officials often delegate to the healthcare professional the tasks of determining how much and what types of services are needed. An allocation from taxes and other revenues, such as "user fees and licenses," is then allocated to the public health enterprise (Legislative Audit Bureau, 2004). Initially, local government was the major source for the funding of the public health enterprise. In the early days, the major tasks of public health were: (1) the collection and interpretation of vital statistics; (2) sanitation; (3) efforts of communicable disease control, such as immunization and quarantine; (4) maternal and child health; (5) health education; and (6) laboratory services (Shonick, 1995).

An essay reviewing early efforts in public health noted the primary concern surrounding the control of communicable disease and the coordinated public health efforts to use sanitation methods to resolve centuries-old health issues:

> When Sir John Simon initiated the modern public health movement in London three quarters of a century ago his primary task was the elimination of the masses of accumulated filth which kept alive the pestilences of the Middle Ages. When General Gorgas undertook the task of making safe and feasible the building of the Panama Canal he was in the same way confronted with problems that were primarily those of environmental sanitation. The removal of excretal wastes, the purification of sewage, the protection of water supplies and the elimination of conditions which permit the breeding of insect carriers of disease—these are always and everywhere the first tasks for the public health expert; and in the early phases of the public health movement in any country it is natural to visualize public health primarily in terms of sanitation.
>
> There is still much to do in this most fundamental branch of public health. That terrible scourge of the Middle Ages, typhus fever, was only held in control during the war by a systematic and organized attempt to destroy the louse which carries the parasite of this disease; while the infection of bubonic plague, the black death of the Middle Ages, has been spread throughout the world during the past twenty-five years, and is held in check only by a vigorous campaign against the rats, ground squirrels, and other rodents which harbor the germ of this peculiar pestilence. The control of malaria, which takes a heavy toll of strength and vitality from the populations of our southern states and is estimated to cost the nation over $100,000,000 a year, is one of the mightiest tasks which confronts the sanitarian, but a task which, as the demonstrations conducted by the International Health Board have made clear, is easily within the range of practical accomplishment, by systematic drainage and other measures taken against the mosquitoes which carry the germs of this disease. Malaria is with us always, but there are many maladies which, like yellow fever, arise from endemic foci in certain particular regions of the globe, and thence spread wherever the

steamship and the railroad train can carry their inciting causes. Of recent years the bold idea has suggested itself of undertaking an offensive against these primary endemic foci of disease without waiting until the invaders cross our own national boundaries. In this way General Gorgas has carried the war against yellow fever into the enemy's own country at Guayaquil, and an organized campaign against such disease on a basis of world cooperation, perhaps through the agency of the International Red Cross, is full of promise of achievement in the future (Winslow, 1920).

Public health financing also addresses whether the allocated amounts are sufficient to keep the society healthy. If the amounts are not sufficient, modifying the allocation plan or raising additional sources of revenues may be necessary. Sometimes the additional revenues are in the form of taxes. At other times it is up to the legislature to make some difficult reallocation choices. Many an election was won or lost by the candidate's reallocation plan (Aidt et al., 2007).

Currently, expenditures for public health services are in excess of $10 billion for all states. Public health expenditures average approximately 3% of total state spending on health services (the majority of expenditures are through the state-administered Medicaid programs). A recent review of state health spending revealed that public health expenditures ranged from 0.6% to 6.4% of total state health spending. In actual dollars, this represents a range of $5.3 million (South Dakota) to $1.7 billion (California) in fiscal year (FY) 2003 (Milbank Memorial Fund, 2005).

PRINCIPLES OF HEALTH ECONOMICS

Public Health Funding Sources

There are four major sources of funding local health departments: local taxes, state grants, federal grants, and fees for service (Wallace & Kohatsu, 2008). There have been significant shifts in the portion coming from each area throughout the 1990s and into the current decade. In 1992, local revenues accounted for only 34% of funding; however, by 2000 this amount had increased to 44% (Wallace & Kohatsu, 2008). During this same time period, the contribution of state revenues shrank from 40% to 30%, while federal funding also decreased from 6% to 3%. Fees for ser-

vice increased slightly over time from 17% to 19% of local health department budgets (Wallace & Kohatsu, 2008).

With an allocation model in hand, public health managers need to determine the source of revenue—that is, where the money will come from. Many public health students have the misconception that funding just appears almost magically from government.

In the 19th and 20th centuries, the scope of what the public health enterprise was required to do became more defined. With the encouragement of the federal government in the late 1980s, financing of the public health enterprise became more standardized and was supported by federal government agencies. By 1998, then, the major sources of money were federal funding, state general funding, and other state funding sources, including fee-for-service revenues. The Milbank Memorial Fund has been tracking the percentages of contribution from each source to state public health funding. **Table 6-1** reveals that an increasing level of federal funding has reached a plateau of just over 50% of public health–related expenditures.

Organized public health efforts on a federal level trace back to 1798, when President John Adams signed the Act for the Relief of Sick and Disabled Seamen into law. Up until 1798 there were marine hospitals scattered throughout port cities on the East Coast, which the law formalized into a network. The hospitals were under the administration of the newly created Marine Hospital Service (MHS). The service was responsible for providing medical care to merchant seamen, especially those suffering from illness and disability.

The new United States borrowed the funding mechanism from England, which understood the importance of maintaining seamen's health. The English funded their programs by taxing seamen's wages each month and included both merchant and Royal Navy seamen. The MHS received funding primarily from a tax of 20 cents per month from seamen's wages. The funds were meant to pay for the services that seamen needed such as medicine, physician care, and room and board. The funds were also meant to help fund the expansion of the program into other port cities.

TABLE 6-1 Direct Public Health Expenditures

Source	FY 1998	FY 1999	FY 2000	FY 2001	FY 2002	FY 2003
Federal funds	47.3%	46.8%	51.2%	50.8%	53.6%	52.7%
State general funds	28.7	30.1	32.0	31.6	23.4	23.1
Other state funds	23.9	23.1	16.8	17.6	21.5	24.1
Undesignated source	0.1	0.1	—	—	1.5	—

Source: Milbank State Health Care Expenditure Reports, 2001, 2003, 2005.

As the service grew, so grew the need for medical services. The service buckled under the stress of the demand and raised taxes to 40 cents per month. The MHS was forced to place restrictions on the system in the form of limiting seamen to four months of care. Seamen with chronic or incurable conditions were outright excluded from receiving care.

Yet the tax increase could not keep pace with demand, so in 1884 the MHS changed the taxation scheme. Instead of taxing seamen's wages per month, a tonnage tax on cargo entering ports via ships was put in place. This financing method was used until 1906, when taxes were no longer the source of funding. Instead, Congress appropriated funds to the service. The program's source of funding was significant in that it was one of the first taxes levied in the nation, and it was also the first medical insurance program.

Federal Government Financing

Over the years the federal government has taken on an increasing role in the financing of public health. These federal programs ensure that some of the basic public health services and programs are available throughout each state, district, and territory of the United States. The two largest healthcare programs are Medicare[1] and Medicaid.[2] Although they do not

---

[1]Authorized by Title XVIII of the Social Security Act, Medicare is the nation's largest health insurance program. In 2006, Medicare provided medical services to 43.2 million beneficiaries and paid claims totaling $402 billion. The Centers for Medicaid and Medicare Services (CMS), an operating division of the Department of Health and Human Services (HHS), administers the Medicare program. Medicare benefits are divided into four parts: (1) Part A consists of inpatient hospital care, skilled nursing facility care, qualified home health care, and hospice care; (2) Part B includes physicians' services, outpatient hospital services, treatment for end-stage renal disease, laboratory services, durable medical equipment, certain elements of home health care, and other medical services and supplies; (3) Part C, the Medicare Advantage program, includes traditional health maintenance organizations, preferred provider organizations, and private fee-for-service plans; and (4) Part D offers beneficiaries an outpatient prescription drug benefit through private plans that contract with Medicare.
Medicare: Thousands of Medicare providers abuse the federal tax system (GAO-08-618). Washington, DC: U.S. Government Accountability Office, 2008.

[2] Title XIX of the Social Security Act is a federal and state entitlement program that pays for medical assistance for certain categories of low-income adults and children. This program, known as Medicaid, became law in 1965 and is jointly funded by the federal and state governments (including the District of Columbia and the territories). Medicaid is the largest source of funding for medical and health-related services for America's poorest people. More than 50 million persons enrolled in the Medicaid program in fiscal year 2006. According to CMS, total outlays for Medicaid (federal and state) in FY 2006 were approximately $324 billion, of which about $185 billion was paid by the federal government.
Medicaid is jointly funded by the federal and state governments. The federal government shares in a state's Medicaid service costs through a matching formula. The federal matching rate for the cost of services provided to Medicaid beneficiaries is related to a state's per capita income, and in federal fiscal year 2006 ranged from 50% to 76%.
Medicaid: Thousands of Medicaid providers abuse the federal tax system (GAO-08-17). Washington, DC: U.S. Government Accountability Office, 2007.

---

fund state and local offices of public health, the programs advance the health of the population, and many Americans benefit from their programs.

With this basic knowledge of public health financing, the general theory of health economics follows. At its most basic definition, *economics* addresses the choices a society makes about how it uses its resources. *Health economics* addresses the choices a society and its individuals make about health care. Remember that in a capitalist society, a force behind these choices is the advancement of the increased success of the firm as indicated by increased profit, stock prices, and even employee job satisfaction.

Economics and Modeling of Public Health Systems

Economics is concerned with the way in which resources are allocated among alternative uses to satisfy human wants. Economics helps us understand the nature and organization of our society, the arguments underlying many of the great public issues of the day, and the operation and behavior of government agencies and private organizations. What do these terms mean? *Human wants* are the things, services, goods, and circumstances that people desire. Wants vary greatly among individuals and over time for the same individual. Some people like improved health status; others want enhanced wages. An individual's desire for a particular good during a particular period of time is not infinite, but in the aggregate, human wants seem to be insatiable. Besides the basic desires for basic health, food, shelter, and clothing, which must be fulfilled to some extent if the human organism is to maintain its existence, wants arise from cultural factors. For example, society, often helped along by advertising and other devices to modify tastes, promotes certain images of the "full, rich life"—these images frequently entail the possession and consumption of certain goods and services. *Resources* are the things or services used to produce services and goods that can be used to satisfy wants. Economic resources are scarce, while free resources such as air are so abundant that they can be obtained without charge. The test of whether a resource is an economic resource or a free resource is price: economic resources command a nonzero price, but free resources do not.

Economics involves the utilization and management of scarce resources. The challenge for public health professionals is to carry health promotion and education technology on one shoulder and the will and imagination to carry the financial burden to perform services with limited resources on the other. How well public health professionals and politicians work together determines whether we experience the bad or good side of market forces. The efficiency of public health systems to guide resources with an "invisible hand" to the right place at the right time involves three components: technical, economic, and allocation efficiency. *Technical efficiency* (also called productivity) refers to the relationship between input and output, irrespective of cost. If one cannot reduce the amount of input and still produce the same amount of output, then maximum technical efficiency has been achieved. In a public health clinic context, for example, inputs might be full-time-equivalent employees, and outputs would be patient visits. *Economic efficiency* refers to the relationship between inputs and cost. When an episode of care is provided at the minimum possible cost, there is economic efficiency. *Allocative efficiency* in health care involves determining which of the inputs that can be used to allocate resources would be least costly for achieving an improved level of output (health status). A health production function is necessary to describe the relationship between a combination of inputs and the resulting output.

The use of these three measures of efficiency can be seen in a public health case study from West Africa. The goal in the production of better health is the reduction of maternal mortality. In Sierra Leone, women have a 1 in 8 chance of dying in childbirth during their lifetime. In developed nations with national health insurance by contrast, the lifetime chance that a woman will die in childbirth is about 1 in 10,000. The rate is even better, 1 in 17,000, in France, Sweden, and Japan. So, how do we reduce the maternal death rate in Sierra Leone? Sierra Leone has a population of 6.4 million people with five gynecologists and 59 other physicians. At the cost of training two additional physicians, the nation could train 100 midwives or 100 traditional birth attendants. We could also build better roads to get the expectant mother to the clinic or hospital. Local village elders in parts of Sierra Leone passed a law requiring all women to give birth at a clinic or face fines of about $10, which is $3 more than the clinic fee. This is an example of setting up negative economic incentives. Wealthier nations have the finances to set up positive incentives—for example, mothers-to-be in France receive a $1,500 voucher if they attend six prenatal visits. The French improved their maternal death rate after implementing this incentive in 1981. By contrast, the United States has a maternal death rate that is 3.3 times higher than that in France (World Health Organization [WHO], 2009).

Cost-effectiveness analysis and cost-benefit analysis have been applied in many preventive, diagnostic, and treatment contexts. Over the past decade, methods have improved for prospectively collecting better data sets and incorporating intangible life valuations into the calculations for weighing benefits against costs. Further cooperation among clinicians, economists, and epidemiologists is a healthy trend. For example, political scientists are prone to argue over valuation in dollars, reflecting a basic misunderstanding of the trade-off concept and the need to combine and compare benefits and

costs in comparable units (Goldie, Kim, & Myers, 2008). In population health terms, if society funds obsolete programs for tuberculosis control that have fewer benefits than costs, the society is made poorer by the venture. The World Health Organization (2008) reports that tuberculosis (TB) was diagnosed in 9.2 million more people, almost exclusively in the developing world, and 1.7 million people died from it. The WHO reports that it is cost-beneficial to provide a new, rapid test for TB that can provide results in as little as two days. Fighting the TB epidemic will require not just newer and more effective drugs, but also better ways to detect the disease and a renewed commitment to expanding existing TB treatment programs.

In addition to evaluating small-ticket, low-price programs for efficiency and effectiveness, researchers also look at the most expensive technologies. Economic evaluation of new or expensive technologies has become a central issue in the public debate about healthcare costs. Historically, the growth in technology has stimulated a concomitant increase in the numbers and salaries of healthcare employees. Physicians and economists frequently express their hope that these expensive technologies are partially justified by their quality-enhancing properties. Sometimes, expensive new technologies can be cost saving (e.g., a kidney transplant); in other cases they are not (Shousboe and Taylor, 2007).

The objective of *cost-benefit analysis* is to maximize net benefits (benefits minus costs, appropriately discounted over time). *Cost-effectiveness analysis* is for ranking preferred alternatives for achieving a single goal or specified basket of benefits. Cost-effectiveness analysis is not easier to perform than cost-benefit analysis if multiple varieties of benefits are specified (person-years, work-loss days, reduced angina), except that in doing cost-benefit analysis, the intangible benefits must be valued in commensurate dollar terms. Operationally, ethical questions can be raised if the benefits and costs accrue to different social groups. For example, a clinic scheduling system that minimizes wasted time for the physician through multiple overlapping appointments might be a net benefit of a few hundred dollars per physician at the expense of many more dollars of patient time. Secondly, a poor nation's urge to build very large clinics or hospitals may be driven by economies-of-scale concerns, but if this increases patient travel time and lost wages (indirect costs), the better alternative may be smaller-scale facilities in each village.

Increasingly, we must justify the cost of public health programs in an era of barebones budgets. We must put the public focus on the production of health. Medline Research Service does not list the word "health" in its index. In a teaching hospital, there is no such thing as a healthy patient. As John Freymann (1998) has observed, a healthy patient is one who has not been sufficiently worked up at a high cost. Come to a teaching hospital as a Medicare patient with the complaint of "stiff hands in the morning," and you may be sent to Rheumatology for a workup to discover Lupus in 1 case per 2,000 screened. In the interest of allocation efficiency, we need to place more emphasis on public health and primary care.

In this section we list and describe several of the more common measures of health status that health economists among other public health researchers use.

Measures of Health Status

Historically, a country's health status was measured by life expectancy. The long-standing measure, however, is giving way to newer gauges of health status (Bleichrodt & Filko, 2008).

- QALY: Quality-adjusted life years calculate life expectancy adjusted for quality of life, where quality of life is measured on a scale from 1 (full health) to 0 (dead).

  QALY = Utility × Probability × Increased life expectancy

- DALY: Disability-adjusted life years combines years of life lost (YLL) through premature death (before 82.5 years for a woman and before 80 years for a man) plus years lived with the disability (YLD).
- DALE: Disability-adjusted life expectancy separates life expectancy into good health years and years lived with the disability. While DALE is estimated to exceed 60 years in half the countries in the WHO, it is less than 40 years in 34 countries.

Quality-Adjusted Life Years (QALY)

QALYs are the gold standard for most cost-effectiveness studies published since 1989. Singer and Younossi (2001) used QALYs as their benefit outcome measure for a cost-effectiveness study of screening for hepatitis C. The analysis does not support the widespread screening for hepatitis C among asymptomatic average-risk adults. The cost-effectiveness results were most sensitive to patient awareness of quality-of-life concerns. Screening was preferred when more than half the patients tested positive for hepatitis C actually initiated treatment, or if the annual progression to cirrhosis was greater than 2.5%.

Different patient populations will have varying levels of cost effectiveness. Vijan's (2001) analysis of colon cancer screening tests revealed incremental cost effectiveness from $20,000 to $300,000 per QALY saved. Cost of colonoscopy and proportion of cancer arising from polyps affect cost effectiveness. In all screening studies, recommendations should be tailored to varying compliance levels in different practice settings. The example concerning hypertension at the end of this chapter is a classic example of this point.

Health education has a major role to play in enhancing maternal and child health outcomes. The locus for education can be the family and the pharmacist. In Asia, fast-growing scales of over-the-counter oxytocin, an injectable hormone that is used to stanch postpartum bleeding and speed labor, will kill if administered incorrectly. The solution has been to educate the pharmacists to educate the family as to when to administer the drug. Blute (2000) analyzed the cost effectiveness of microwave thermotherapy in patients with benign prostatic hyperplasia and concluded it exhibited the highest five-year utility value (4.4 QALYs) compared to medical treatment. The incremental cost per QALY gained was $39,000 for thermotherapy compared with medical therapy. Many nations cannot afford this level of fiscal support. The World Bank considers three types of evaluations for comparing alternatives: cost minimization, incremental net benefit, and incremental cost effectiveness (Eastaugh, 2004).

Many services that are effective are not covered by insurance. Why are proven preventive services underinsured? Even in the event that preventive services provide cost savings, the gains may be so far in the future or the elasticity of supply in the industry may be so high that insurance companies are unable to reap any benefits. One of the problems with preventive screening examinations is that the cost of treating false-positive results, along with adverse psychological effects, might outweigh the benefit of detecting a disease in its early stages (Eastaugh, 2003).

It is not necessary to conduct economic analysis and randomized clinical trials on every new technology—and certainly not on most existing ones. The uncontrollable economic pressures for efficiency are apt to result in more careful economic analysis. Some of these studies will severely disrupt the conventional wisdom. For example, Russell (1995) studied a number of preventive programs and concluded that society's total healthcare costs increased (i.e., most prevention was a cost add-on, not a cost-saving investment). Investments that cost very little on a per-person basis become very costly when applied on a national basis. Russell cited the example of a blood pressure check, which is very inexpensive on an individual basis, but becomes very costly when applied to 30 million people.

In any health economics study, clinicians and economists must work together to define a population goal of benefits, that is, a basket of benefits (e.g. reduced mortality, reduced morbidity, for a defined population). Magid, Douglas, and Schwartz (1996) did this by comparing treatment strategies for women with uncomplicated cervical chlymadial infections: (1) initial therapy with doxycycline, 100 mg orally twice daily for 7 days (estimated cost, $5.51); (2) initial therapy with azithromycin, 1 g orally administered in a single dose (estimated cost, $18.75). In a sensitivity analysis (varying the assumptions across a range of variables), the azithromycin strategy prevented more major complications but was more expensive than the doxycycline strategy, but doxycycline effectiveness was greater than 0.93. In a multivariate sensitivity analysis combining 11 parameter estimates selected so that the cost effectiveness of the doxycycline strategy would be maximized relative to that of the azithromycin strategy, the azithromycin strategy resulted in fewer complications but was more costly. The incremental cost effectiveness, the cost to stop the development of a complication, was $521 per additional major complication prevented.

Methods of Economic Analysis

Public and political disenchantment has been high with economists who provide narrow definitions of direct benefits and ignore the limitations of their very crude databases. A valid and reliable economic analysis must (1) make the evaluation as complex as necessary, (2) assign values to resources that reflect their opportunity costs, (3) avoid zero counting of resources, and (4) avoid double counting of resources. The typical accounting costs of billed charges or incurred expenses define cost too narrowly for the economic analyst (Gold et al., 1999). Confusion frequently exists when members of the medical profession attempt to perform a cost analysis. For example, the cost to society of not improving car safety with airbags is substantial. In population health terms, if we do not have airbags, more accident victims will be dead on arrival. As another example, if we do not reduce the incidence of HIV, the disease burden on the public will expand significantly.

In the arena of cost-effectiveness analysis between medical treatment and surgery, surgeons frequently omit from the analysis those who die during surgery to make surgery look better relative to medical treatment (Eastaugh, 2003). The tendency is to go far afield in counting benefits and to neglect some costs, such as the pain of surgery or the overhead costs of the operating room. Cost of cash expenditures is defined too narrowly. True cost to society can only be measured in opportunity cost terms, or in terms of the value of the benefit sacrificed to obtain it.

Estimating the economic burden of a disease involves the measurement of *prevalence*, the assessment of effect on health status and on others' well-being, and the eventual quantification of direct and indirect costs associated with these effects. For example, the cost of alcohol abuse is an estimated $114 billion in 2008. More than half of the alcohol abuse burden on the economy resulted from lost economic production ($61 billion); $27 billion was generated from direct healthcare service costs; and $26 billion resulted from motor vehicle accidents, fires, crime, and other less tangible effects (Eastaugh, 2008).

A number of sources of uncertainty exist for making economic decisions. The first source of analytical uncertainty results from incomplete mastery of available knowledge in medicine coupled with the fact that medicine is in a constant state of flux and revision. A second source results from limitations in current medical knowledge (Bendavid, Young, & Katzenstein, 2008). Human immunodeficiency virus-1 (HIV-1), HIV-2, Lyme disease, Legionnaires' disease, and eosinophilia-myalgia syndrome were characterized only recently, and new disease entities are discovered every year. The third source of uncertainty, derived from the first two, is the difficulty in distinguishing between ignorance and the limitations of current medical knowledge—that is, the fear of the untaught versus the fear of the unknown.

The critical point to convey to the reader is that cost-effectiveness analysis and cost-benefit analysis are taking their appropriate positions more and more frequently in the evaluation (prediffusion) stage prior to the marketing decision. The rationale of this emerging public policy is that the costs (in lives and in dollars) of forgoing economic and efficacy evaluation might often be much greater than the costs of a well-designed evaluation. One "consumerist" benefit of increasing reliance on economic evaluation is that it must force those in power to be explicit about (1) valuation-of-life biases (across social class) in cost-benefit calculations and (2) the resource cutoff level utilized in cost-effectiveness analysis (Eastaugh 2002).

Net Present Value Analysis: Discounting

The public health manager who is not an economist frequently misunderstands that inflation is only one part of the rationale for discounting. Even if all benefits were adjusted for the projected rate of inflation, discounting would still be necessary to account for the social rate of time preference. Discounting makes allowance for the time value of money—that is, if you have a benefit in dollars in year 4 and a cost in dollars in year 2, you need to place all dollars in current baseline year 0, dollars. Therefore, all dollars of benefit and all dollars of cost are brought back into baseline year 0 dollars by utilizing the *discount rate*. It presumes that benefits and costs are juxtaposed and measured in commensurable dollar units at a single given discount rate (Jena & Phillipson, 2008). Choice of a discount rate is of no consequence for a short-lived program with benefits and costs concentrated within one to two years.

Selection of the rate of discount is a crucial parameter in most net present value calculations. A prediction that technology will become more cost-increasing in the future argues for selection of a lower discount rate in order to make lifesaving more valuable in future years. This viewpoint is supported by the suggestion that technology is reaching a state of diminishing returns, where even an optimistic 50% reduction in the three leading causes of death (cardiovascular disease, cancer, and motor vehicle accidents) would add less than one year of life for people aged 15 to 65. There are three basic varieties of discount rates: (1) the corporate discount rate if the private sector borrowed the funds, (2) the government borrowing rate on bond issues in the marketplace, and (3) the social discount rate to enable programs and procedures with benefits far in the future to prove more acceptable. Public health decision makers only use the social discount rate. The social discount rate (Pigou, 1920) is probably used most often because of the strength of its intergenerational equity argument. For example, a $25 million one-shot project in 2009 with a payoff of $75 million in the year 2030 has a positive net present value only if the discount rate is 6% or less. The typical social discount rate is on the order of 3% to 4%. The discount rate is vital to balance benefits and expenses over many years—that is, the expenses are frontloaded but the benefits can last for decades.

Applications of Cost-Effectiveness Analysis

The purpose of cost-effectiveness analysis is to identify the preferred alternatives. Physician preoccupation with survival probabilities must not preclude measurement of quality-of-life factors in performing a cost-effectiveness analysis. Cost-effectiveness analysis still requires that intangible factors be measured; however, they do not have to be valued. Typically, the search for preferred alternatives involves comparisons of less-invasive treatment. Further research is needed as to the timing and content of the best means of promoting cost-effective clinical decisions. For example, in Africa malaria is a major public health problem. To enhance population health, we must provide one mosquito net to sleep under for each family member, plus two fishing nets. If we do not provide fishing nets, the family uses the mosquito nets to fish, tearing the net, and reducing malaria control effectiveness.

Patient education is a major issue in health services delivery. For example, we can teach diabetics to use pocket insulin-dosage computers to enhance independence and self-esteem and save money by reducing the rate of hospital admissions among brittle diabetics. Often what is less costly is better for the patient: use a $19 pulse oximeter to get the same basic information as arterial blood gases, thus saving $75 and reducing the discomfort for the patient (as long as acidosis or CO_2 retention is not suspected). The style of medical practice is moving toward cost-effective clinical decision making. Most nephrologists do not order a metabolic workup for the first kidney stone. Pulmonary specialists order spirometry, rather than expensive but more complete pulmonary function testing, for the preoperative chronic emphysema patient. Emergency medicine physicians have come up with five rules to cut costs:

(1) not X-raying everyone with low back strain, (2) not ordering Chem-7s and CBCs on young healthy patients with a day or two of gastroenteritis, (3) getting a chest X-ray rather than rib films on young patients with rib fractures, (4) not getting an EDIVP on every young healthy patient with clinical evidence of kidney stone, and (5) dipping urine as a screening test rather than using microscopy on every urine sample.

Technology assessment proceeds in sequential stages. Physicians dominate the first stage of analysis, examining short-term safety and descriptive analysis (e.g., does the new technique or procedure yield improvements?). Statisticians dominate the second stage of technology assessment with a middle-term study of efficacy utilizing randomized controlled clinical trials. Diagnostic efficacy studies report sensitivity and specificity (Lee, 2008). Economists and policy makers dominate the third stage of technology assessment: clinical cost effectiveness (is it less costly than the alternative options at achieving a prescribed package of "effects," e.g., X percent less pain or Y percent less morbidity?) and long-run cost-benefit (does the ratio of benefit to cost exceed 1, counting all costs and benefits to society?). Because cost-benefit analysis should include intangible benefits (e.g., pain reduction) to be comprehensive, it is necessary to shadow-price patients' willingness-to-pay preferences regarding a given technology.

Some programs have obvious cost-savings potential, like smoking cessation for mothers. Lightwood (2000) reports that an annual drop of 1 percentage point in smoking prevalence would prevent 1,300 low-birth-weight live births and save $21 million in direct medical costs in the first year of the program; it would prevent 57,200 low-birth-weight infants and save $572 million in direct medical costs in seven years. However, most of public health is not so clear-cut in the quick return on the healthcare intervention.

Economic evaluations must take into consideration the difference between efficacy and effectiveness. *Efficacy* is the maximum possible benefit, often achieved with controlled trials, and *effectiveness* is the actual decrease in disease achieved when the intervention is applied over a large, nonhomogeneous population (Meltzer, 2001).

The goal of public health education programs is to apprise service providers of the appropriate use of tests, procedures, and treatment options. Educational efforts come in a number of formats, offered in combination, including didactic lectures, restructuring of order forms, cost feedback, concurrent or retrospective protocol review, and other retrospective medical record audits. The didactic course approach typically makes four basic points: (1) work cost effectively (e.g., home health care or ambulatory surgery); (2) perform a cost-benefit assessment of the case management alternatives; (3) avoid unnecessary, outmoded, or duplicative procedures; and (4) encourage preventive and health promotion activities. On this last point, health promotion can do more than reduce future illness; it can also reduce duration of stay, patient anxiety, and complications. The essence of a cost-effectiveness analysis is the measurement of the incremental cost and effects that result from choosing one strategic option over another (e.g., influenza vaccine for healthcare workers versus no vaccine) (Detsky & Kaupacis, 2007).

Cost-Benefit Analysis

The objective of cost-benefit analysis (CBA) is to maximize net benefits (benefits minus costs, appropriately discounted). Successful preventive medicine programs in terms of dollar benefit are child immunization, smoking prevention, lead reduction, and water fluoridation. Immunization, for example, saves $8.50 in direct medical costs for every dollar spent on childhood immunization. Smoking prevention efforts over the past 30 years are estimated to have saved 33 million person-years of life. Lifetime medical expenses of smokers are put at $46,000 for men ($11,000 more than for nonsmoking men) and $68,000 for women smokers ($13,000 more than for woman nonsmokers) (Eastaugh, 2004).

Lead poisoning has also been reduced as a major source of childhood disease. From 1988 to 1997, there was a 58% reduction in presentation of children with high levels of lead in their blood (currently 700,000 children). The reason for this drops includes federal initiatives to end the use of lead in gasoline, lead solder in the seams of food cans, and lead-based paints in homes. It is estimated that reducing the level of environmental lead has improved cognitive function in children to the degree that it has increased lifetime earnings by $1,147 per mg/dL difference in blood-lead levels per child. In addition, a cost analysis of removing lead from paint estimated a net benefit of $63 billion in reduced medical costs (Eastaugh, 2003).

Dental health should not be overlooked in population health assessment. The decline in dental caries during the past 40 years as a result of water fluoridation has been such that half the children in the United States are caries-free. During an individual's lifetime, the dentistry costs of carious teeth might exceed $1,000, but water fluoridation costs about $0.12 per person per year.

To measure the costs and benefits of a specific program, it is necessary to express net value in fiscal terms so that benefits can be weighed against the costs. The 1999 National Oceanic and Atmospheric Administration (NOAA), co-chaired by Nobel Prize winners Kenneth Arrow and Robert Solow, renewed interest in willingness-to-pay (WTP) methods for valuation of benefits. The NOAA issued new regulations promoting the use of contingent valuation studies for assessment of damage to natural resources. Eastaugh (2003) offered a contingent valuation study measuring WTP for treatment of patients with von Willebrand's disease. Median WTP for treatment of this disorder was $1,500 or $3,500, depending on how the initial bid was structured. Regression analysis shows that income, education, and a category rating scale for health status were significant in predicting WTP. The adjusted annual WTP was $2,178. WTP surveys may be increasingly useful for health technology assessment. Starting point bias in how the bids are structured must be recognized, and the potential bias of the results can be reduced by random assignment of 10% of the sample to one-tenth of the starting bids. Therefore, one-tenth of the respondents would anchor an initial bid at $5,000, one-tenth at $4,500, and so on, with one-tenth at the lowest initial bid of $500. There is need for further testing of the WTP and contingent valuation methods. The casual reader may incorrectly suggest that WTP is only needed for cost-benefit studies. WTP is also needed for cost-effectiveness studies to assess whether a cost per QALY is low or high, and whether a price per QALY is necessary (Bishai, Sindelav, & Ricketts, 2008).

The gains and losses of providing public health programs apply not only to the person whose treatment is in question, but to the rest of us as well. One way public health managers do this is through CBA. In economic sectors in which competitive markets fail to exist, such as the healthcare or water resource sectors, CBA aims to do what supply and demand forces accomplish in competitive markets. The price system will not equalize marginal benefits and marginal costs if market failure exists, as it always does in public health. One criterion of choice is maximization of the ratio of benefits to costs, discounting the numerator and denominator to present-day dollars. Alternative programs (or procedures or services) are then ranked by cost-benefit ratios, and the programs with the highest payoff ratio are selected until resources are exhausted or until the ratio equals 1. This approach is equivalent to maximizing net present value in a budget constraint. A third, but outmoded, decision criterion is to support a project if the internal rate-of-return criterion exceeds the predetermined discount rate. The internal rate-of-return criterion can lead to different resource decisions from the net present value criteria if programs are of different sizes or have varying time horizons (Negrin & Polo, 2008).

If a technology is found to be the most cost-effective alternative, then the next question is whether it is cost beneficial. For example, Acton (1973) first evaluated which of five program alternatives was most efficacious and which was most cost effective in reducing deaths from heart attacks. He followed valuation of life and intangible benefits to assess whether the benefits made the program worth the costs to society. One obvious advantage of CBA is that it leads to a positive (go) or negative (no-go) net present value for the procedure being evaluated and does not require a cost-effectiveness cutoff level to decide whether a project can be completed within the resource constraints. However, many more complete cost-effectiveness analyses than CBA are performed, because intangible benefits pose difficulties with valuation, and the choice of a discount rate is simpler in cost-effectiveness evaluations (Eastaugh, 2002).

If a technology is found to be cost beneficial, the only question left is whether the risk is socially acceptable for public financing of the service. Society may have some preference for the social classes that are to face an unacceptable risk, even if it is known in advance that the total risk is insufficient to make the benefit-to-cost ratio less than 1. Safety, as a measure by risk analysis, is a relative concept. No test or therapy that provides any benefit has ever been completely safe. Public health workers, like all professionals, have learned to live comfortably with the reasonable notion that we must forgo some safety to achieve any net benefit.

In the American context, two basic truths seem apparent. First, society should not be oversold on prevention and health promotion as a strategy to slow (or reverse) the inflation in national health expenditures. If health officials oversell their programs as a cost-saving vehicle, the inevitable disillusion will cause excessive additional cuts in public health programs (i.e., the backlash against such programs). Second, prevention might not save money, but such programs can often be justified in terms of worthwhile investment in improved quality of life (Eastaugh, 2004). Keeping people happy is expensive, but in the minds of most citizens, quality of life is something worth paying for.

Measurement of Intangible Benefits

Valuation, or placing a dollar value on health status or pain reduction, is not an easy task. Valuation is not a consideration in competitive business markets, because marginal benefit is assumed to be equal to price. However, when prices fail to exist (water resources) or price is deemed a defective measure of value (health services), an attempt is made to impute value, placing what economists call a *shadow price*. Shadow-price values can be imputed by asking individuals what they would be willing to pay for relief from pain, grief, discomfort, and disfigurement. Let us consider a population health issue such as how frequently should we screen for breast cancer. For example, if a year of life is valued by a willingness-to-pay measure of $28,000, and a woman would sacrifice a year of life to avoid losing her breast(s), this suggests a shadow price of $28,000 for a mastec-

tomy (Acton, 1973). In this situation, Acton suggested that the additional costs for a few more drugs would bring the average shadow price, adding in the cost of grief and worry, to about $31,000. Often the analysts can only identify the need to shadow-price an intangible benefit. For example, one intangible that is difficult to shadow-price is the benefit of restored fertility capacity that follows a successful kidney transplant.

The shadow-price concept can also be applied to arrive at quality weights for adjusting the value of additional years of existence. We can use an analogous-disease approach to measure the willingness-to-pay value of escape from early manifestations of syphilis by the proxy disease psoriasis and from the last manifestations of syphilis by the proxy of terminal cancer cases. Direct data acquisition for "unstigmatized" medical conditions like cancer and psoriasis was more easily accomplished than working directly with syphilis victims. Economists must work with physicians to develop proxies and weighting schemes for capturing the multiplicity of dimensions of healthcare outputs. Inappropriate priorities might be set if survival probabilities are not integrated with quality-of-life factors.

The Harvard study by Keeler (1999) offers a good assessment of quality-of-life considerations after coronary artery bypass surgery. Quality-of-life outcome measures include pain at rest, pain with minimal activity, pain with mild activity, pain with strenuous activity, and no pain. Quite predictably, a potential surgical patient places a higher utility value on no pain if he or she avoids exercise. A utility function to value outcomes was specified as a function of lifestyle and life expectancy. The data are highly subjective, but reliance on imperfect analysis provides more insights than analytical nihilism. A Rand Corporation analyst (Keeler, 1999) reported that the lifetime subsidy by the average citizen to the sedentary lifestyle person is $1,900. Lifestyle choice is a critical issue for many medical decisions.

Cost-effectiveness analysis is more frequently completed when it is recognized that intangible benefits need only be estimated, not valued. Cost-effectiveness analysis requires only that all benefits be expressed in commensurate units so that the cost of achieving a specified level of benefits might be minimized. In one study at George Washington University, we found that many women at risk of premature delivery were not getting corticosteroids, which improve the lung function of prematures babies (Eastaugh, 2003). Based on this evidence, the use of corticosteroids tripled. The benefit? A 9.9% drop in deaths of low-birth-weight babies and millions of dollars in savings by avoiding the cost of treating complications. Cost-effectiveness analysis is not any simpler than cost-benefit analysis if multiple varieties of benefit are specified (e.g., in lives, years, or pain), except that in doing cost-benefit analysis, we must also value intangible benefits.

Opinions on Risk Are Not Mathematical

We do not live in a safe world. Risk analysis is complex in public health. Cutting one risk typically creates another. For example, if the Russian Republic were to convert the inferior 80% of its nuclear generating capacity to coal, over the next four decades the increased traffic from coal trucks, mining accidents, and pollution-induced disease would kill 1.8 million citizens. Many citizens fear nuclear power because unknown fears outrank familiar ones. Breathing or drinking vodka are things a person is familiar with. Consuming radiation from a nuclear accident or eating and drinking dioxin and polychlorinated biphenyls are not familiar experiences. The standard dosage of cosmic radiation at sea level is 2,000 times more dangerous to human life than residing in a home 20 miles from an American nuclear power plant. One round trip from New York to Los Angeles has 200 times more risk than living next to a U.S. nuclear plant.

Risk assessment is one of the critical issues in population health assessment. Risk assessment models are typically simplistic. The U.S. Environmental Protection Agency (EPA) uses a linear standard risk assessment model; for example, if 20 out of 1,000 rats get cancer from eating two bowls of dioxin a day, the EPA assumes that half a bowl per day would kill only five rats. Sliding down the dosage response curve, the EPA assumes that at 0.006 picogram per day, one human in a million would die of cancer. Linear models that assume that damage is in exact proportion to dosage are seldom accurate representations of the situation. The more accurate nonlinear models report risk as a decaying exponential function; therefore, government officials in Australia and Canada allow safe doses of dioxin at rates 300 to 500 times the U.S. threshold (standard). Moving to a dioxin standard that is 10 times tougher than the Australian threshold would save the American people $1.1 billion in cleanup costs, according to California analyst Dennis Paustenbach at McLaren Environmental Engineering. Formaldehyde has the classic "hockey-stick" dose response curve: it is safe until the dosage exceeds 10 parts per million, but at 15 parts per million, 50 percent of the animals get cancer. The American aversion to risk is not based on mathematics or common sense. Moderate content of PCBs in the daily diet has 90% to 98% less risk than eating two tablespoons of peanut butter per day. Peanut butter can contain mold-producing aflatoxin, but we do not ban peanut butter because it is an all-American food.

In economics, an *externality* (or external defect) directly affects the welfare of other people or firms, resulting from the use of a commodity by some other consumer or firm. Producing pollution (e.g., acid rain or secondhand smoke) that harms me is an example of a negative externality. The major-ity of the class having vaccinations that enhance the population of the group is an example of a positive externality. If an individual does not receive a vaccination, but all the other group members are vaccinated, the individual is called a "free-rider."

Avoiding a little risk can sometimes create a larger long-term risk. For example, 1960 data suggested that when whooping cough vaccine is given to 1 million children, 95 will have serious reactions (and a few will die). In the United Kingdom, parental pressure caused the National Health Service to withdraw the vaccination requirement. Whooping cough deaths soared, and the requirement was reinstated.

If small risks are often overlooked, large risks of catastrophic expense are highly unpredictable. Society should treat catastrophic medical expenses like the demand for firefighting equipment. No one stands outside a burning building and demands out-of-pocket payments to do the job of firefighting. This argues for collectivizing the burden of catastrophic medical expenses, either in the manner of the United Kingdom (free care) or through public insurance (Eastaugh, 2008).

WILLINGNESS TO PAY

Federal and state governments promote mandates to make things happen (e.g., reduce pollution or disease). Government uses willingness-to-pay surveys to assess health benefits. The *willingness-to-pay* (WTP) *principle* in normative economics states that the value of something is simply measured by what people are willing to pay for it. Economists generally agree as a canon of faith that each person best knows his or her own interests. Cost-benefit analysis has to operate within the bounds of the individual's deficient information base, congenital optimism, or hypochondria, and to accept the expressed consumer preferences as a more relevant measure of benefits than the expert opinions of an educated elite. Experts' presumption that the public is unable to properly assess its interests may be foiled on two counts: (1) The observation that people respond in a biased emotional fashion may be irrelevant for policy-making purposes if the bias is unsystematic, because the extremes will cancel each other; and (2) We could make the same argument that the public cannot understand the technical details necessary to purchase calculators, cameras, cars, and stereos. The public does not have to understand all the details, as long as a free flow of information creates some small cadre of amateur consultant friends to help guide consumer choice behavior. Providers are improving their capacity to plug patient utilities into the decision analysis; survey researchers are more sensitive to elderly respondents; and development of a quality-of-well-being scale has even extended to acquired immune deficiency syndrome, arthritis, and cystic fibrosis (Eastaugh, 2004).

The early WTP study most often cited was done on a sample of 100 Boston residents by Acton (1973). Acton's most publicized question involving public attitude toward risk reduction and heart attacks reads as follows:

> Let's suppose that your doctor tells you that the odds are 99:1 against your having a heart attack. If you have the attack, the odds are 3:2 that you will live. The heart-attack program would mean that the odds are 4:1 that you live after a heart attack. How much are you willing to pay in taxes per year to have this heart-attack program which would cut your probability of dying from a heart attack in half (i.e., the chances are 2 per 1,000 you will have a heart attack and be saved by the program this year)?

The median response was $56, suggesting that 200 people would chip in $28,000 to save the life of the group members in the coming year. The scenario is reasonable because most health programs are risk-reduction efforts. One might also note that a small change in the question, reducing the risk to 0.001, increases the median imputed value of a life saved to $43,000. Both of the two aforementioned questions emphasize the individual's situation. When Acton posed the question in probabilistic terms, focusing on the 10,000 people living around a hypothetical respondent, the medical amounts were reduced by approximately 50% for equivalent risk-reduction levels.

The WTP approach can be criticized on the grounds that life is probably valued much higher for identified individuals than for members of a hypothetical population. Consumers and physicians tend to value identified individual lives more than statistical anonymous forgone lives, yet physicians are often criticized for placing a substantially higher value on identified individuals than society, with its limited resources, can afford to place on the average citizens.

The success of the WTP approach may be somewhat limited, because the methodology is fraught with problems. However, to paraphrase Winston Churchill, the approach is terrible unless you stop and compare it to the alternatives (your discounted wages are your worth). The WTP technique generates troublesome questions, but not nearly as troublesome as assuming that a group is merely worth the amount its members can earn, or assuming that the political fiat is superior to economic measurements and evaluation. Those who favor political fiat over analysis may pause to count the number of times pork barrel projects consumed resources that could have gone to education and public health.

Willingness to pay has an analogue called willingness to accept (WTA). If you are a duck or chicken farmer in China, you have a higher WTA risk from avian flu than the general public. We have asked the maximum amount that an individual is willing to pay for a program or service, but we could also ask the minimum amount that an individual is willing to accept to forgo the service or program. If future economic conditions prompt a contraction in the social welfare programs (e.g., Georgia's in 2008), more economists may be surveying the WTA issue. The divergence between WTP and WTA survey results may be an example of the Will Rogers rule: the public knows more about limits than the economists or the politicians. Consumers make mistakes because they are provided with imperfect information, so individuals' WTP is sometimes underestimated (e.g., vaccinations) and other times overestimated (e.g., Laetrile).

Valuation problems tend to plague many public health analysts. Subjective questions concerning valuation and effectiveness are largely a product of the values and occupation of the respondent. Young educated physicians might value a life at $10 million, but the average voter sets a value 28% lower. In 2008, the Bush administration valued a life at $7.22 million. If the average American will accept a 1 in 10,000 chance of death for $722, then the value of one life must be 10,000 × $733, or $7.22 million.

A central dilemma that the economic analyst faces is the unsubstantiated thesis of ever-improving technology—that is, the assumption that any evaluation will be obsolete when completed because medical science improves so quickly. Yet another problem faced by the analyst attempting to do a prospective study is refusal by the physicians to pursue randomized controlled trials if any hint of inferiority among the alternatives can be raised as a red herring to prevent the experiment. Difficult decisions will need to be made more and more frequently concerning the allocation of scarce resources.

Hypothetical WTP Survey Techniques

One central research issue that Arrow (1978), Eastaugh (2003), and others have identified is the timing of a willingness-to-pay evaluation. The issue is whether respondents should be surveyed *ex ante* under a veil of ignorance concerning their future disease prognosis, or whether the survey should be done *ex post* on patients with more information concerning the prognosis for themselves or members of their socioeconomic group. The problem to be considered is one of response bias, because the *ex post* WTP responses will surely be highly inflated—that is, the answers will be high because the opportunity costs of those remaining dollars, given the shortened amount of time, are low to the individual about to die. Obviously, people who have a fatal disease may answer with a higher WTP response than the average citizen. However, with some chronic conditions this assertion appears to be false—that is, the general population overstates the burden of all illness more than the actual victims do. In other words, *ex post* WTP responses by victims should be adjusted downward because their WTP is based, in part, on their increased chances of fatality. For example, the WTP for fire protection by storeowners on the currently unaffected half of a burning city block would certainly be higher than the WTP of the average storeowner in the city. A rational public service cannot be planned based on the preferences of respondents undergoing a catastrophe.

Utility preferences for attributes the consumer values (e.g., pain reduction, mobility enhancement) need not be linear or independent of wealth. Risk aversion and risk preference can be observed to change over time in the same individual or concurrently in the same person under different hypothetical situations. In valuing lifesaving activities for statistical lives, the wording of the question is a very important issue. Consider an example outside the context of health care. If the government wants to help American companies with "incentives," 68% of the public favor the program; but if the government wants to provide "subsidies," then 60% are against it, even when the programs are exactly equivalent. Economists have discovered a number of elegant techniques to elicit consumer WTP preferences, but questionnaires have yet to be utilized for making substantial resource allocation decisions. The most obvious practical problem with hypothetical WTP measures is that the questions could be considered too unreal to be treated seriously by some respondents. One way to avoid this problem is to present a plausible scenario that concerns a risky situation that has been reported on the news.

As with all surveys, the best WTP questionnaires would avoid the use of value-laden wording. For example, people do not like to be asked the question, "How much is your grandfather worth?" More reasonable answers will be given if 1,000 people facing a 0.002 chance of dying next year are asked, "How much would you pay to reduce your risk by 0.001?" In other words, these 1,000 individuals are asked their willingness to pay to save one statistical life, which will not be identified until next year. It is common knowledge that society places very high values on identifiable lives facing a high probability of death or disfigurement. The media frequently report a high level of psychic benefit accruing to the population following a heroic rescue attempt or an attempt to aid an identified child. For example, individuals seem to experience more psychic benefits as a group in supporting the identifiable March of Dimes Poster Child than in supporting Medicaid for multi-institutional charity hospitals. Arrow (1978) was the first to observe that individuals jump to help one 6-year-old identified life, but few shed a tear or write a check if a tax shortfall causes fa-

cilities to deteriorate, thereby causing a barely perceptible statistical increase in preventable deaths.

The most basic problem with WTP valuation is that the appropriate database to make estimates with any adequate range of confidence does not exist. Three subsidiary problems concern, in many cases, (1) the lack of public health worker input in identification of the subtle side effects that should go into the analysis, (2) the lack of appropriate behavioral science survey instruments, and (3) the lack of an appropriate population to survey. As an example of this last problem, in doing a WTP analysis of benzene cleanup activities, which people should be selected for the survey—workers heavily exposed to benzene, all workers, or all those who bear the burden of the cleanup? Should people with a given disease be sampled while hospitalized, should potential candidates for the disease be surveyed, or should all citizens be queried? How is the survey instrument to be written if researchers are unsure whether benzene starts to bring about significant increases in the incidence of leukemia by x percent at prolonged exposure levels of 40 parts per million, 20 parts, or 1 part?

Another problem with WTP consumer preference surveys is that the results may not be very stable over time. The public may express a lower WTP for avoiding a relatively higher and familiar risk (like automobile fatality) than a lower but unfamiliar risk. Some individuals get alarmed over the prospect of a nuclear accident, yet they tolerate much higher risks in their daily lives.

In addition to valuing life, consumer preference surveys can assist in the selection of an optimum therapy. Most progressive physicians have recognized, at least in theory, which treatment decisions should attempt to incorporate patient values into the decision. However, most clinicians are untrained in the disciplines of economics and behavioral decision theory and cannot scientifically survey patient preferences. The sensitive clinician attempts a "quick-and-dirty" approach to get some handle on patient values by asking, "Would you rather have short-term certain survival for, say, 5 years or gamble on an operation that has a low probability of death but offers an additional 20 years of life expectancy?" Physicians are increasingly coming to respect the value of asking such questions.

Health education, which has been assailed by skeptics, is a popular current example of a new approach to improving the effectiveness of medical care. **Table 6-2** presents the results of a cost-benefit comparison of four approaches to increasing patient compliance to antihypertensive medications.

The study sample for Table 6-2 included 402 patients randomly assigned to experimental and control groups (Eastaugh, 2004). The emphasis of the study concerned the efficacy of utilizing a triage process, whereby patients were subdivided

TABLE 6-2 Simple Cost-Benefit Comparisons of Triage Options Versus the Option Not to Triage in Achieving Improved Medication Compliance Among Hypertensives

Option	Triage	Type of Patient	IHC	Education Intervention(s)	Cost-Benefit Ratio
1	Yes	High level of depression	65–26	Family reinforcement (FR)	2.2
2	Yes	Medium level of depression	58–33	FR + message clarification	1.15
3	Yes	No depression	65–33	FR + message clarification	1.33
4	No	All patients	60–32	FR + message clarification	1.24

into groups more predisposed to benefit from a given health education approach. The benefits of the triage method for achieving medication compliance clearly outweigh the cost only in the case of the highly depressed patients (24.3 percent of the sample), as defined by responses to five of the seven items used in the depression scale questionnaire. The cost-benefit ratio for this group (2.2) compares favorably with the average cost-benefit ratio of 1.24 for hypertension control for persons in the age range of 35 to 65 (option 4). In other words, triaging only the highly depressed subpopulation (24%) and providing family member reinforcement is more cost beneficial than giving everyone the special health education intervention. Previous studies demonstrating a cost-benefit ratio in the 1.1 to 1.3 range may not stand the test of time in claiming a statistically significant ratio above the 1.0 level when ap-

plied to a larger population or to a nonexperimental population that will be less susceptible to the Hawthorne effect. Individuals are known to change their behavior more dramatically under experimental conditions due to the mere fact of being under concerned observation.

CONCLUSION

The willingness-to-pay approach to cost-benefit analysis is one elixir that will not make decision making any easier, but at least the process could increase consumer input and illuminate the assumptions that currently prevail. Policy makers must take note that public health is most effective when it prevents problems. It is better to put a fence at the top of the cliff than an ambulance at the bottom.

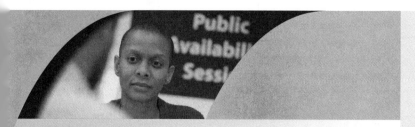

Discussion Questions

1. Who finances public health services in the United States?

2. What historical factors led to the current finance situation?

3. Can it be changed?

4. The percentage of U.S. gross domestic product needed for health services hovers around 17%. This is reportedly the largest percentage of any Western country. With your new understanding of public health finance and health economics, describe at least four finance or economic reasons that contribute to this large value.

5. Should there be a cap on public health spending?

6. How do we finance health disasters such as the H1N1 virus?

7. Are quality measures good indicators of sound economic policy?

REFERENCES

Acton J. Evaluating Public Programs to Save Lives: The Case of Heart Attacks. *Rand Corporation Report R-950-RC.* Santa Monica, CA: Rand Corporation; 1973.

Aidt TS, Veiga FJ, Veiga LG. Social Science Research Network. *Election Results and Opportunistic Policies: An Integrated Approach.* October 12, 2007. NIPE Working Paper No. 24/2007. http://ssrn.com/abstract=1022292.

Arrow K. Risk Allocation and Information: Some Recent Theoretical Developments. Paper presented at: Geneva Papers on Risk and Insurance, 1978; Geneva, Switzerland.

Bendavid E, Young S, Katzenstein D. Cost effectiveness of HIV monitoring strategies. *Archives of Internal Medicine.* 2008;168(17):1910–1918.

Bishai D, Sindelav J, Ricketts E. Willingness to pay for drug rehabilitation. *Journal of Health Economics.* 2008;27(4):959–972.

Bleichrodt H, Filko M. New test of QALYs when health varies over time. *Journal of Health Economics.* 2008;27(5):1237–1249.

Blute M. Cost-effectiveness of microwave therapy. *Urology.* 2000;56(6):981–987.

Detsky A, Laupacis A. Relevance of cost-effectiveness analysis. *JAMA.* 2007;98(2):221–225.

Eastaugh S. Cost-effectiveness in home healthcare. *Managed Care Quarterly.* 2002;1:41–49.

Eastaugh S. Willingness-to-pay. *International Journal of Technology Assessment in Health Care.* 2003;16(2):706–711.

Eastaugh S. *Healthcare Finance and Economics.* Sudbury, MA: Jones and Bartlett; 2004.

Eastaugh S. Healthcare reformation: Lessons from other nations. *Harvard Health Policy Review.* 2008;9(1):49–57.

Freymann J. The public's health paradigm is shifting. *Journal of General Internal Medicine.* 1998;4(4):319–329.

Gold M, Siegel J, Rusell L, Wernstein M. *Cost-Effectiveness in Health and Medicine.* New York: Oxford University Press; 1999.

Goldie S, Kim J, Myers E. Cost-effectiveness of cervical cancer screening. *Vaccine.* 2008;24(3):5164–5170.

Jena A, Phillipson T. Cost-effectiveness analysis and innovation. *Journal of Health Economics.* 2008;27(5):1224–1236.

Keeler E. The external cost of a sedentary lifestyle. *American Journal of Public Health.* 1999;79(8):975–981.

Legislative Audit Bureau. *Best practices report: Local government user fees.* Madison, WI: State of Wisconsin; 2004.

Lee R. Future costs in cost-effective analysis. *Journal of Health Economics.* 2008;27(4):809–818.

Lightwood J. Health and economic benefits of smoking cessation: low birth weight. *Pediatrics.* 2000;104(6):1312–1320.

Magid D, Douglas J, Schwartz J. Doxycycline compared with azithromycin for treating chlamydia. *Annals of Internal Medicine.* 1996;124(4):389–399.

Meltzer D. Addressing uncertainty in medical cost-effectiveness analysis. *Journal of Health Economics.* 2001;20(1):109–128.

Milbank Memorial Fund, National Association of State Budget Officers, the Reforming States Group. *1998-1999 State Health Care Expenditure Report* 2001.

Milbank Memorial Fund, National Association of State Budget Officers, the Reforming States Group. *2000-2001 State Health Care Expenditure Report* 2003.

Milbank Memorial Fund, National Association of State Budget Officers, the Reforming States Group. *2002-2003 State Health Care Expenditure Report* 2005.

Negrin M, Polo F. Incorporating model uncertainty in cost-effectiveness analysis. *Journal of Health Economics.* 2008;27(5):1250–1259.

Pigou A. *The Economics of Welfare.* London: Macmillan; 1920.

Russell L. *Is Prevention Better Than Cure?* Washington, DC: Brookings; 1995.

Shonick W. *Government and Health Services: Government's Role in the Development of U.S. Health Services 1930–1980.* New York: Oxford; 1995.

Shousboe J, Taylor B. Cost-effectiveness of bone densitrometry. *JAMA.* 2007;298(6):629–637.

Singer M, Younossi Z. Cost effectiveness of screening for hepatitis C virus in asymptomatic, average-risk adults. *American Journal of Medicine.* 2001; 111(8):614–621.

Vijan S. Which colon cancer screening test. *American Journal of Medicine.* 2001;111(8):593–601.

Wallace R, Kohatsu N. *Public Health and Preventative Medicine.* New York: McGraw-Hill; 2008.

Winslow CEA. The untilled fields of public health. *Science.* 1920;51(1306): 23–33.

World Health Organization. *World Health Reports 2009.* Geneva: WHO; 2009.

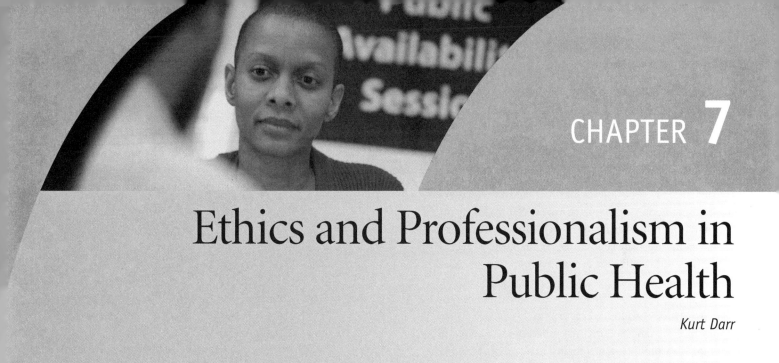

CHAPTER 7

Ethics and Professionalism in Public Health

Kurt Darr

INTRODUCTION

This chapter sets out the role and effect of ethics in the practice and professionalism of public health. After a short exposition of the relationship of law to ethics, this chapter addresses the need for public health managers to appreciate the importance of their organization's culture and values, the role of their own personal ethic, and the effect of both on the quality and efficacy of the services they provide. The chapter concludes by identifying and discussing some major ethical issues that affect public health organizations and those who manage them, including conflicts of interest, fiduciary duty, gratuities, consent, resource allocation, staffing, quality of services provided, research, politicization of public health, and generally providing the structure and support so that those served by the organization receive safe, effective services and so that their autonomy is enhanced.

LEARNING OBJECTIVES

After reading this chapter, the reader will be able to:

1. Define ethics and its relationship to law.
2. Understand the role and content of a personal ethic.
3. Recognize the importance of an organization's mission, vision, and values.
4. Apply moral philosophies and ethical principles relevant to public health.
5. Understand and apply professional codes of ethics in public health.
6. Identify ethical issues in public health and minimize their negative effect.

BACKGROUND

Philosophers define ethics as the formal study of morality. Sociologists see ethics as the mores, customs, and behavior found in a culture. For physicians and healthcare professionals, ethics means meeting the expectations of their profession and society and acting in certain ways toward patients. Managers in public health must see their value system—their ethic—as a special charge and responsibility to those served by the organization, the organization's staff, to themselves and the profession, and, ultimately, to society. In doing their work, managers in public health must ask themselves the question of normative ethics: "What ought I (we) to do (in this situation)?"

Both ethics and law arise from a society's value system (moral framework). Ethics is at once a source of the law and a function of it. *Ethics* can be defined as the study of standards of conduct and moral judgment. The ethics of a profession is the group's principles or code—its self-imposed value system. The *law* is a system of principles and rules for human conduct that arises from a society's value system, is prescribed or recognized by society, and enforced by public authority. This definition fits both criminal and civil law.

Managers in public health (and health services, generally) are held to a higher standard. This likely results from their role as public servants and their association with the healing professions of medicine and nursing—from whom much is expected. And, it is also likely to be an expectation that none of those served by such an organization should have their trust breached—the trust inherent in the intimate, emotional, and vital relationships established in the process of protecting the public's health and in delivering health services.

HEALTHCARE ETHICS

Relationship of Law to Ethics

Democratically derived laws generally reflect the majority's views of justice and fairness. Some in society may consider a law unjust or immoral and risk or invite punishment by breaking it. Contemporary examples are the widespread recreational use of marijuana and engaging in civil disobedience to protest government or private actions deemed morally wrong.

Ethics and law diverge in many ways, and what is lawful may be judged by some (or many) to be unethical and what is unlawful may be judged to be ethical. In most permutations, the law is the minimum performance expected in society. Professions demand that their members obey the law, but simultaneously hold them to a higher standard. Thus, a profession's code of ethics requires that members act in ways different from other persons in society.

Henderson's models (1982) identify the relationships of law and ethics. **Figure 7-1** shows the succession of events that results in the public scrutiny of an organization's decisions and a judgment as to whether they are legal, ethical, or both. The judgment is necessarily retrospective, despite management's

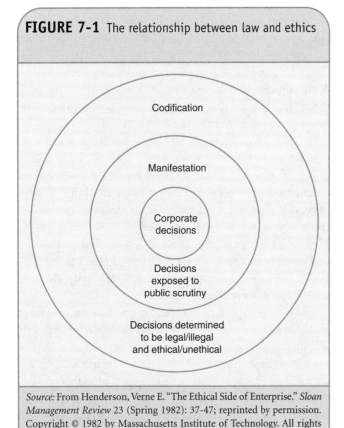

FIGURE 7-1 The relationship between law and ethics

Codification

Manifestation

Corporate decisions

Decisions exposed to public scrutiny

Decisions determined to be legal/illegal and ethical/unethical

efforts to predict the effects of decisions. It is common to find managers deliberating the effect and implications of their decision making both internally and externally. The model suggests the difficulty of knowing whether those who eventually judge the decision will consider it legal (e.g., law enforcement officials) or ethical (e.g., a profession or the public). This adds uncertainty to organizational decision making. Predicting an action's legality is often easier than predicting whether it will be judged ethical (fair or right).

Figure 7-2 shows the combinations of legal, illegal, ethical, and unethical factors that are involved in an organization's decision making. Decisions made in Quadrant I are ethical and legal and easily identified: managers who obey the law are acting ethically and legally. Quadrant II includes decisions that are ethical, but illegal. Professional codes of ethics typically require that obeying the law is the minimal level of performance for ethical conduct. Such an expectation means that only compelling moral justification may exculpate an illegal act by a manager. An example is to disregard a law because obeying it will cause a significant injustice for a staff member or someone served by the organization. Quadrant III includes decisions that are unethical but legal. This quadrant is often reflected in a profession's code of ethics that requires performance more demanding than the law. Examples include failing to take *all* reasonable steps to protect members of the public from harm or managerial self-aggrandizement to the detriment of those served by the organization. Quadrant IV includes activities that are both illegal and unethical. Examples are easy. Professional codes of ethics typically require that members obey the law; actions that break the law are both illegal and unethical. Deliberately failing to meet fire safety regulations, embezzlement, or knowingly filing a false government report lie in this quadrant.

The Manager's Personal Ethic

Each of us brings to our professional lives a set of moral values—a personal ethic. This personal ethic is the result of values imparted from sources such as family and friends; religious training; self-study, education, life experience, and introspection; and professional codes of ethics. A personal ethic can incorporate both positive and negative values. It defines who the person is from a moral standpoint.

The personal ethic is likely to evolve over time. It should, however, be understood and evaluated prospectively and reflect the qualities of coherence (fits with experience), comprehensiveness (addresses a broad range of ethical issues), and consistency (similar ethical problems will be solved similarly). Many public health practitioners are drawn from the health professions of medicine and nursing, both of which

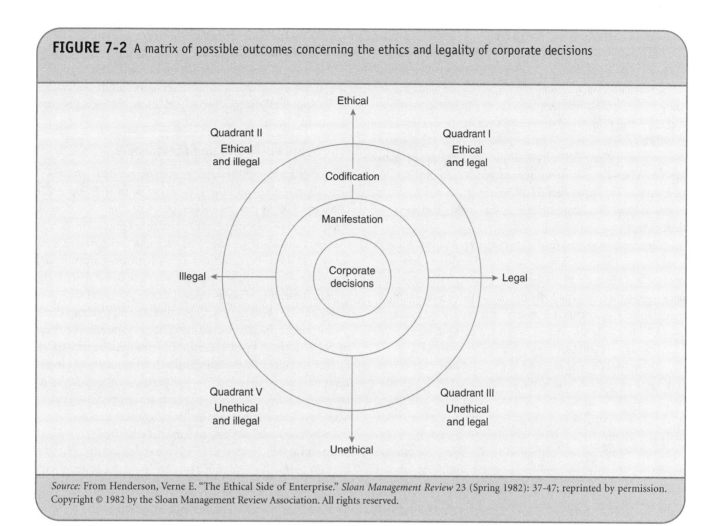

FIGURE 7-2 A matrix of possible outcomes concerning the ethics and legality of corporate decisions

Source: From Henderson, Verne E. "The Ethical Side of Enterprise." *Sloan Management Review* 23 (Spring 1982): 37-47; reprinted by permission. Copyright © 1982 by the Sloan Management Review Association. All rights reserved.

bring to their work a rich tradition of attention to ethics. Instruction in ethics may have been included in their professional training.

Academic preparation in medicine and nursing provides training in analysis, patterns of logical thought, and sequential reasoning, all of which are valuable qualities in developing a personal ethic and solving ethical problems. Lack of a clearly defined personal ethic will result in relativistic ethical problem solving. Use of *ethical relativism* is undesirable because it fails to incorporate a values framework that should be present in every public health activity. Specifically, ethical relativism lacks coherence, comprehensiveness, and consistency. It is difficult to overstate the importance of a well-developed personal value system—the personal ethic. In addition, the academic preparation sensitizes public health practitioners to the managerial and clinical ethical issues that they are likely to encounter and provides a framework for analysis and solving ethical problems.

The net result is that public health practitioners have been socialized to understand that they are entering a field in which they manage a social enterprise with business dimensions, rather than a business enterprise with social dimensions. This fact in itself makes the public health organization and those working in it unique and more closely resembling eleemosynary organizations such as not-for-profit hospitals than other types of service organizations. Persons served by public health organizations have a unique relationship with it. This relationship is expressed through a level of trust in the organization and implicitly its management that is rarely found in the non–health service industry.

Organizational Philosophy and Values

The concept of organizational philosophy and values was introduced in Chapter 2. It bears restating that, for better or for worse, all organizations have an identifiable culture—its shared, unique values. Organizations should perform periodic values audits, which are similar to financial audits, to identify and describe the values present in the culture. This approach "discovers" those values. Rather than discovering the values of the culture, however, it is more typical that senior managers develop a statement of values that they *may* hold themselves or that they think *should* be those espoused by the organization and those working in it. The statement of values that results may or may not reflect the true culture (values) of the organization. In fact, the statement may have little to do with its actual values. A pretty plaque hanging in the lobby that lists values alien to the organization's culture makes a mockery of the concept of shared values.

Culture (and values) can be affected over time, but doing so is slow, almost glacial. Managers must lead in this evolutionary effort. They *must* model all the values that are desired—those present and those to which the organization aspires. Failing to model the desired values, but asking staff to do what managers are unwilling to do themselves, will do naught but lead to cynical, uninvolved staff. Leading by example is essential.

The values desired must be key to, and provide the context for, all organizational activities. For example, these values must provide the criteria for all staff recruitment, screening, hiring, evaluation, and retention. Failure to measure candidates against the framework in which they will work invariably leads to mismatches of context and staff. The consequences will be higher costs and unnecessary and counterproductive levels of dissatisfaction, or worse. In terms of the organization's services and how they are provided, its values should be inviolate. This is to say that, despite the demands of users, the organization can maintain its integrity only if it refuses to act in ways inconsistent with its values. It must be true to itself. Public health organizations may face pressures from elected officials to act in ways inconsistent with their values. Resisting such pressures reinforces the need for managers to have a well-developed, clearly enunciated personal ethic and for the organization to have a well-defined value system that is followed in all activities. All policies, procedures, and rules of the organization must reflect this value system as well.

The culture must support the philosophy and associated values that the organization considers important. Congruity is essential, lest the culture (or important parts of it) be unsupportive. Incongruity will result in conflict, discontinuity, and waste (Nelson, Weeks, & Campfield, 2008). A major and continuing challenge for the public health manager is to establish and enhance a culture that incorporates the organizational philosophy and its values.

Mission, Vision, Values

The *mission statement* sets out why the organization exists. The *vision* identifies the direction in which the organization wishes

to go—its aspiration, or what it seeks to become. As noted, *values* are derived from and are part of the organization's philosophy and should be embedded in and reinforced by the culture. If the organization is to succeed, its culture and values must support efforts to achieve its mission and make progress toward its vision.

Organizational Values and the Manager

Questions arise as to the need for congruence between the organization's values and the personal ethic of staff, especially managers. Simply put, the values (personal ethic) of staff at all levels should be congruent with that of the organization. Ideally, the congruity is one-to-one. While this may be unlikely, it is essential that the cores of the two value systems are compatible and consistent. Only by achieving a high level of congruence is the organization able to live its values by developing a strong, pervasive culture. Assuming staff members have a generally compatible value system (personal ethic), the organization's culture must be taught to them and must be reinforced by the actions of all, but especially those in leadership positions. Managers must not only understand the organization's culture, but must attempt to move the values it reflects from where they are to where it is desirable that they be. This suggests the need for managers to have a well-developed personal ethic that they understand and as well as values they espouse and reflect in everything they do personally *and* professionally. A strong culture, with clearly defined and shared values will drive from it those whose interests and actions are contrary. This in itself is a worthy goal. High levels of cultural conformity may stifle innovation, but this risk can be overcome in other ways, such as including innovation as an identified, important value in the culture.

Some managers may bristle at the prospect of having their personal lives subject to scrutiny and open to rebuke. History and experience have shown, however, that managers of public health organizations reify that organization. Little distinguishes the two in the public's eye. Public health managers who embarrass or scandalize their organization and, consequently, the governing body, should polish their résumés. For better or worse, in organizations that serve the public in the health field, one's personal life is directly and inextricably connected to one's public life.

Applicable Moral Philosophies

Moral philosophies assist us in knowing what we should do—*normative ethics*. The unique role of public health organizations means that ethical issues have legal dimensions and that legal issues have ethical aspects. Capable managers see both. The dynamic relationship between ethics and law that was described earlier is sometimes synergistic, sometimes antagonistic. Each affects and is affected by the other. The law is the basic framework of society and the context for application of ethics in the field of public health.

Moral Philosophies

Teleology, deontology, and natural law have found extensive application in Western societies. Two other moral philosophies, virtue ethics and casuistry, have experienced a revival and are considered, as well. These five moral philosophies provide a basis to study morals (ethics), provide a framework for a personal ethic and an organizational philosophy, and help determine the moral rightness or wrongness of an action.

Teleology *Teleology* is derived from *telos*, Greek for "end." The most prominent moral philosophy using this concept is utility theory; its followers are utilitarians. The underlying premise is that the moral rightness or wrongness of an act or decision is judged by whether it brings into being more good (utility) or ungood (disutility) than alternative decisions. Classical utilitarianism's most prominent proponent was the English philosopher John Stuart Mill (1806–1873). Utilitarians have no independent right or wrong to guide them. They look at the consequences of an act—the "good" as independent of the "right." Utilitarians are sometimes called consequentialists because they judge actions by their consequences.

Utilitarianism is divided into act utility and rule utility. *Act utility* assesses each decision and determines its consequences when judging moral rightness or wrongness. Act utilitarians judge each action independently, without reference to preestablished guidelines (rules). They measure the amount of good, or (nonmoral) value, brought into being and the amount of evil, or (nonmoral) disvalue, brought into being or avoided by acting on a particular choice. Each person affected is counted equally. This suggests a strong sense of objectivity. Act utilitarianism receives no further attention in this discussion because it is episodic and incompatible with deriving the ethical principles needed for an organizational philosophy, a personal ethic, or professional codes of ethics.

Rule utility is formal. It assesses courses of action (or nonaction) and measures their consequences—the amount of (nonmoral) good or ungood produced. The morally superior course of action must be taken, even though it may not produce the most good (least ungood) in a specific application. Utility theory is the basis for cost-benefit analysis. A crude summary statement describing utilitarianism is "the end justifies the means."

Deontology Deontology is based on the presence of an independent right or wrong. It does not consider consequences. *Deontology* is derived from *deon*, Greek for "duty." The best-known proponent of a duty-based moral philosophy was the German philosopher Immanuel Kant (1724–1804). Briefly,

Kantian deontology asserts that the end (result) is unimportant because human beings have duties to one another as moral agents and these duties take precedence over consequences. For Kant, an act is moral if it arises from good will and if, therefore, one acts from a sense of duty. The Kantian test of morality is whether the act can meet the categorical imperative, which requires that we act in accordance with what we wish to become a universal law. The *universal law* is that what is right or wrong for one person is right or wrong for everyone, in all places and at all times. According to Kant, an action is right only if it can be universalized without violating the equality of human beings. For example, Kantians see it as logically inconsistent to argue that a terminally ill person should be euthanized (actively causing death) because this is saying that life can be improved by ending it. Deontology may be summarized as never treating human beings simply as a means but rather always as an end (Kant, 1959). Another summary of deontology is to practice the Golden Rule—do unto others as you would have them do unto you.

The work of a contemporary American philosopher, John Rawls (1921–2005), extended Kantian deontology. In *A Theory of Justice*, Rawls (1971) used elaborate philosophical constructs to develop the elements of a social contract among free, equal, self-interested, and rational persons. He reasoned that such persons would reject utilitarianism and select instead the concepts of right and justice as necessary to the good. Rawls argued that rational, self-interested persons, knowing nothing of what they are or will become, would develop a system (1) that maximizes liberty and (2) where social and economic inequalities would be to everyone's advantage. Any redistribution of goods and services would be done in an egalitarian (equal) manner. He argued that because we might be in the least position, we would want to maximize the minimum position that a person could be in—because it could be us.

Natural Law *Natural law* states that ethics (morality) must be grounded in a concern for human good, and is, therefore, teleological (consequential). Natural law is based on Aristotelian thought as interpreted and synthesized with Christian dogma by St. Thomas Aquinas (ca. 1225–1274) (Bodenheimer). It assumes a natural order in relationships and a predisposition among rational persons to do, or refrain from doing, certain things. Because human beings are rational, we are able to discover what we should do, and in that attempt we are guided by a partial notion of the eternal law that is linked to our capacity for rational thought. For example, we see that other human beings are like us and are entitled to the same respect and dignity that we want. Because natural law guides what rational persons do, it is the basis for positive law, some of which is reflected in statutes. Natural law contends that the good cannot be defined only in terms of subjective inclinations; rather, there is a good for human beings that is objectively desirable, although not reducible to desire (Arras & Rhoden, 1989). A summary statement of the basic precepts of natural law is that we should "do good and avoid evil."

Casuistry Many historical definitions of *casuistry* are disparaging. Critics argue that it uses evasive reasoning and encourages rationalizations for desired ethical results. Regardless, contemporary advocates see casuistry as a pragmatic way to understand and solve ethical problems. Casuistry is case-based reasoning in historical context. It avoids excessive reliance on principles and rules, which may provide only partial answers and may not guide decision makers comprehensively. Casuistry allows problem solvers to use the concrete circumstances of actual cases and the specific maxims that people invoke in facing actual moral dilemmas (Jonsen & Toulmin, 1988).

At its base, casuistry is similar to the law, where court cases and the precedents they establish guide decision makers. "Cases in ethics are similar: Normative judgments emerge through majoritarian consensus in society and in institutions because careful attention has been paid to the details of particular problem cases. That consensus then becomes authoritative and is extended to relevantly similar cases" (Beauchamp & Walters, 1994, p. 21). For example, hospitals and nursing facilities use casuistry as ethics committees develop a body of experience with various ethical issues.

Both medical and management education rely on cases. This makes it natural to use them in health services, in which traditional ethics problem solving has applied moral principles to cases—from the general to the specific, or deductive reasoning. Modern casuists can profitably copy the classical casuists's reliance on paradigm cases, reference to broad consensus, and acceptance of probable certitude—assent to a proposition, but acknowledging that its opposite might be true (Jonsen, 1986). Greater numbers of cases in public health organizations and a body of experience will lead to consensus and more certainty in charting moral direction.

Virtue Ethics *Virtue ethics* focuses on what makes a good person, rather than on what makes a good action. The practice of virtue goes beyond the law and observing moral rights and duties. Western thought about the importance of virtue can be partially traced to Aristotle. Similar to natural law, virtue is based on theological ethics but without a primary focus on obligations or duties. Like casuistry, it has received more attention, some of which results from a perception that traditional rule- or principle-based moral philosophies, deal inadequately with the realities of ethical decision making. This is to say that virtue ethicists argue that rules are of limited help in solving ethical problems. When there are competing ethical rules or situations to which no rules apply, something more than a coin toss is needed. Here, virtue ethicists claim to have a superior moral philosophy.

Contemporary authors argue that virtue ethics has three levels. The first two are observing laws and observing moral rights and fulfilling moral duties that go beyond the law. The third and highest level is the practice of virtue:

> Virtue implies a character trait, an internal disposition habitually to seek moral perfection, to live one's life in accord with a moral law, and to attain a balance between noble intention and just action. . . . In almost any view the virtuous person is someone we can trust to act habitually in a good way—courageously, honestly, justly, wisely, and temperately (Pellegrino & Thomasma, 1988, p. 121).

In this view, virtuous physicians (or public health managers) are disposed to the right and good intrinsic to the practice of their profession and will work for the good of those being served.

Some virtue ethicists argue that, as with any skill or expertise, practice and constant striving to achieve virtuous traits (good works) improve one's ability to be virtuous. Others argue that accepting in one's heart the forgiveness and reconciliation offered by God (faith) "would lead to a new disposition toward God (trust) and the neighbor (love), much as a physician or patient might be judged to be a different (and better) person following changed dispositions toward those persons with whom . . . [they] are involved" (Carney, 1978).

All people should live virtuous lives, but those in the health professions have a special obligation to do so. Virtuous managers and physicians are not just virtuous people practicing a profession; they are expected to work for the good of those served even at the expense of personal sacrifice and legitimate self-interest (Pellegrino & Thomasma, 1988, p. 116). Virtuous physicians, for example, place the good of their patients above their own and seek that good unless pursuing it imposes an injustice on them or their families, or violates their conscience (Pellegrino, 1994). Similarly, virtuous managers in public health put the good of those served above their own even at the expense of personal sacrifice and legitimate self-interest. Thus, virtuous managers speak out to protect those being served even when doing so risks their continued employment.

Linking Theory and Action

Principles, rules, and specific judgments and actions rely on or are based on ethical theories. Ethical theories do not necessarily conflict; diverse moral philosophies may reach the same conclusion about an action, albeit through different reasoning or the use of varying constructs.

Ethical theories and derivative principles guide development of rules that produce specific judgments and actions. Four principles should guide decisions in public health: respect for persons, beneficence, nonmaleficence, and justice. These principles should be reflected in the organization's philosophy and culture, as well as in the manager's personal ethic.

Respect for Persons

The principle of *respect for persons* has four elements. The first, *autonomy*, requires that one act toward others in a way that enables them to be self-governing. Basically, this is the right to be left alone. It is a negative right—the right to decline unwanted treatment. It can be described, too, as a liberty right—the right to be free from interference. This liberty right is inviolable so long as its exercise does not interfere with the rights of other persons. Exceptions occur in public health. Examples of interfering with others' rights include mandatory vaccinations of school-age children, isolation and quarantine of persons to slow or stop epidemics, and required reporting of certain types of infectious diseases. Here, the rationale is clear and long-established: the law recognizes that individual (liberty) rights cannot be allowed to put society at risk, generally. Autonomy is not a positive or distributive right, which are those granted or guaranteed by an entitlement program.

To choose and pursue a course of action, people must be rational and uncoerced (unconstrained). Sometimes physical or mental conditions cause someone to become nonautonomous. They are owed respect, nonetheless, even though special means are needed to enable them to express their autonomy. Autonomy underlies the need to obtain consent for treatment, as well as the general way in which public health organizations view and interact with those served by it and its staff.

Autonomy is in dynamic tension with paternalism. The Hippocratic oath is antecedent to paternalism in the patient–physician relationship and suggests that physicians should act in their patients' best interests—as physicians judge those interests. Giving autonomy primacy limits paternalism to specific circumstances.

The second element of respect for persons is *truth telling*, which requires managers and staff to be honest in all they do. At its absolute, truth telling eliminates "white lies," even if knowing the truth causes harm to the person learning it. One measure of respect is that we are truthful with one another. Lying to someone is an expression of disrespect. It is Kantian to show persons respect by telling them the truth. Consider the ramifications for public health if the persons served could

not trust those in positions of managerial or clinical authority to tell the truth. Calculating the good and ungood brought into being (the ends) by lying is utilitarian. Loss of trust because of lying would bring into being much more ungood than good. Thus, the morally correct choice for both the deontologist and the utilitarian is to tell the truth.

Confidentiality, the third element of respect for persons, requires managers and clinicians to keep secret what they learn about persons served and others in the course of their work. Legal requirements for case finding and reporting necessitate morally justified exceptions to confidentiality. All in the organization are expected to keep confidential what is learned in the process of delivering services. Ethically (and legally), information can be shared only on a need-to-know basis. Organizations are commonly abuzz with idle chatter, gossip, and unnecessary discussion of clients' (and staff's) circumstances, including unauthorized review of files. These breaches of confidentiality must be stopped because they contravene the values the organization should have.

The fourth element of respect for persons is *fidelity*, defined as doing one's duty or keeping one's word. Sometimes called promise keeping, fidelity requires managers to be respectful of all persons, whether they are being served by the organization, staff in the organization, or others. Keeping one's promises and being faithful in our relationships and interactions not only treat persons with respect, but further the delivery of services (a utilitarian measure).

Beneficence

The second principle, *beneficence*, is rooted in the Hippocratic tradition and is defined as acting with charity and kindness. Contemporary public health applications of beneficence are broader, including a positive duty to the public. Generally, beneficence anchors one end of a continuum, at the opposite end of which is the principle of nonmaleficence, defined as refraining from actions that aggravate a problem or cause other negative results.

Beneficence is comprised of conferring benefits and balancing benefits and harms. The former is well-established in medicine; failing to provide them when one can do so violates an ethical obligation of clinicians. This principle is equally applicable in public health. Modified to be consistent with their role, beneficence applies to managers, as well. The positive duty suggested by beneficence requires the public health organization to do all it can for persons served. There is a lesser, but identifiable duty to aid persons who are potential rather than actual recipients of services. Application of this distinction varies with the organization's mission and vision and with the population served.

The second dimension of beneficence is balancing the benefits and harms of an action. This is the concept of utility, the philosophical basis for cost-benefit and risk-benefit analyses. Utility is but one of several considerations in public health decision making. Its more limited application results from a positive duty to act in the best interests of the person being served because one cannot act with kindness and charity if risks outweigh benefits. Regardless, utility cannot be used to morally justify overriding the interests of persons being served and sacrificing them to the greater good. The positive duty of beneficence requires public health managers and their organizations to do all they can to aid and benefit those being served.

Nonmaleficence

The third principle applicable to managing in public health is *nonmaleficence*. It, too, has deep historical roots in medicine. Nonmaleficence can be defined as *primum non nocere*—first, do no harm. This dictum to guide physicians applies equally to managers in public health. Nonmaleficence gives rise to specific moral rules, but neither the principle nor derivative rules is absolute. For example, it may be appropriate (with consent) to inflict harm (e.g., administer anti-rabies vaccine) to avoid worse harm (e.g., contracting rabies) and appropriate to compromise truth telling if telling the truth would result in significant mental or physical harm to the person(s) being served.

The principle of nonmaleficence also means that managers have duties to staff. Putting staff at unnecessary or extraordinary risk to their health and safety violates a manager's duty to them, even if the result meets the principle of beneficence to persons being served. Balancing benefits and harms also suggests application of the concept of utility.

Justice

The fourth principle, *justice*, is important in managerial decision making such as allocating the organization's resources or developing and applying human resources policies. What is justice, and how does one know when it is achieved? Justice has various definitions. Some definitions require that all persons get their just desserts—what they are due—which supports merit-based decision making. Rawls defined justice as fairness. But how are just desserts and fairness defined? Aristotle defined justice as equals being treated equally, and unequals being treated unequally—a concept common to public policy analysis. Equal treatment of equals is reflected in liberty rights such as freedom of speech for all. Unequal treatment of people unequally situated is used to justify redistribution of wealth through state and federal tax codes. Aristotle's concept of justice is expressed in public health when greater resources are expended for those with greater needs. These concepts of

justice are helpful, but do not solve problems of definition and opinion that are often troublesome for managers. At minimum, managers act justly by consistently applying clear and prospectively determined criteria in decision making.

Summary

Moral philosophies and derivative principles provide a framework to hone and apply a personal ethic to analyze and solve ethical problems. Managers are unlikely to adopt only one moral philosophy. Most will be eclectic in developing or reconsidering their personal ethic. The principles of respect for persons, beneficence, nonmaleficence, and justice are a useful starting point in defining relationships among those being served, managers, staff, and organizations. The principles should be reflected in all of the policies, procedures, and rules used by the organization. The principles may carry different weights and take precedence over one another, depending on the issue. Justice requires, however, that they must be consistently ordered and weighted as similar ethical issues are considered.

ETHICS IN PRACTICE

Codes of Ethics that Affect Public Health Management
In seeking professional status, managers throughout the public and private systems of healthcare services delivery have established and joined professional associations that have developed and adopted codes of ethics. These codes vary in their level of proscription and prescription and the methods of enforcement, but all have the common thread of doing what is in the best interest of those served by the organization—usually defined as the person served.

The codes tend to emphasize respect for persons (autonomy, truth telling, fidelity, and confidentiality), beneficence, nonmaleficence, and justice. Applying these ethical principles widely used in clinical ethical decision making is sometimes strained; nevertheless, they provide a useful starting point that is supplemented as needed by other principles.

The Hippocratic oath was written approximately 2,400 years ago by Greek physicians, one of whom could have been Hippocrates. It continues to be relevant in medical practice, as well as in all relationships between and among the practice of public health and the various relationships that result. The Hippocratic oath includes a philosophy about relationships among physicians and between physicians and patients, and its high standards for physicians continue today. Principles that remain applicable include respect for colleagues, confidentiality of medical information, prohibitions on euthanasia and physician-assisted suicide, and appropriate professional relationships with patients. The oath limits treatment to dietetic therapies—a concept that may be waxing—and prohibits physicians from undertaking surgery, a ban no longer applicable in allopathic medicine. A modern version of the Hippocratic oath was written in 1964 by Louis Lasagna and reflects those portions of the original Hippocratic oath applicable to contemporary allopathic medical practice.

Professional codes of ethics identify expected levels of performance as well as the striving of the profession. They are a means for that profession to communicate expectations to its members. Codes are most effective in guiding behavior of the members of a profession when they include monitoring and the requirement of self-discipline. Expectations must be sufficiently precise in order for the code to provide meaningful guidance to members of the profession, those charged with enforcing the code, and society in general. Codes of ethics must be living documents, guiding professionals who want to do the right thing, but who may be uncertain as to what that is. In this regard, education is an important factor, and education about a profession's ethical code should be part of any continuing executive development program undertaken in that profession.

Codes of Ethics in Public Health

The American Public Health Association (APHA) has no code of ethics, but its website has links to several others that provide ethical guidelines for practice and research in public health. In part, the introduction to the list of websites states:

> Public health practitioners by virtue of our roles have special responsibilities for ethical conduct and ethical practices that go beyond meeting minimum legal and regulatory standards. Our broad range of practice in public health policy; in the delivery of healthcare through programs and services; and, in administration, research, education, social service, business and other related functions is essential to the health and well being of their population and communities. Our roles and functions demand that we conduct ourselves in an ethical manner that emphasizes a population or community-focus, and justifies the public trust (http://www.apha.org/about/Public+Health+Links/downloaded July 15, 2008).

This introductory statement reflects the earlier discussion about the differences between law and ethics. It identifies the need for public health professionals to hold themselves to a standard higher than that set by the law. With or without such expectations, the public is almost certain to hold them to a higher standard. Maintaining the public's trust requires that public health professionals be paragons of virtue in all that they do. Once lost, restoring the public's trust will be difficult, if not impossible.

Ethical Practice in Public Health

The "Principles of the Ethical Practice of Public Health" were developed by the Public Health Leadership Society and published in 2002. The document sets out a list of values and beliefs (assumptions) that underlie public health and provide a context for the 12 principles of the ethical practice of public health that are enunciated in **Table 7-1**. A section following explication of the 12 ethical principles provides explanatory information about each. The ethical principles apply to the practice of public health. It is unclear, however, how and by whom (or what) success (or failure) in meeting them is judged. No attention is paid to the ethical implications of good management and the need to use resources efficiently and effectively. Apparently, these judgments are left to individual managers and the organizations for which they work. Examples of these beliefs and values include the following: humans have the right to the resources necessary for health, humans are inherently social and interdependent, effectiveness of institutions depends heavily on the public's trust, collaboration is a key element in public health, people and their physical environment are interdependent, science is the basis for much of our public health knowledge, and people are responsible to act on the basis of what they know.

Health Education

The Society for Public Health Education has adopted the "Code of Ethics for the Health Education Profession" (2003). The code includes six articles: responsibility to the public, responsibility to the profession, responsibility to employers, responsibility in the delivery of health education, responsibility in research and evaluation, and responsibility in professional preparation. Each of the six is followed by explanatory material about the article. All of the expectations are stated positively. The code requires neither reporting of breaches of the expectations nor is there a disciplinary process for those who fail to meet the code.

Other Guidelines

The ethical guidelines for epidemiological studies are less relevant to the day-to-day activities of most public health organizations. The Council for International Organizations of Medical Sciences, in collaboration with the World Health Organization, has issued the "International Ethical Guidelines for Epidemiological Studies." These guidelines are similar to those required by the U.S. Department of Health and Human Services (HHS) for research involving human subjects. Provisions include ethical justification and scientific validity of epidemiological research involving human subjects; ethical

TABLE 7-1 The 12 Principles of the Ethical Practice of Public Health

1. Public health should address principally the fundamental causes of disease and requirements for health, aiming to prevent adverse health outcomes.
2. Public health should achieve community health in a way that respects the rights of individuals in the community.
3. Public health policies, programs, and priorities should be developed and evaluated through processes that ensure an opportunity for input from community members.
4. Public health should advocate and work for the empowerment of disenfranchised community members, aiming to ensure that the basic resources and conditions necessary for health are accessible to all.
5. Public health should seek the information needed to implement effective policies and programs that protect and promote health.
6. Public health institutions should provide communities with the information they have that is needed for decisions on policies or programs and should obtain the community's consent for their implementation.
7. Public health institutions should act in a timely manner on the information they have within the resources and the mandate given to them by the public.
8. Public health programs and policies should incorporate a variety of approaches that anticipate and respect diverse values, beliefs, and cultures in the community.
9. Public health programs and policies should be implemented in a manner that most enhances the physical and social environment.
10. Public health institutions should protect the confidentiality of information that can bring harm to an individual or community if made public. Exceptions must be justified on the basis of the high likelihood of significant harm to the individual or others.
11. Public health institutions should ensure the professional competence of their employees.
12. Public health institutions and their employees should engage in collaborations and affiliations in ways that build the public's trust and the institution's effectiveness.

review committees; ethical review of externally sponsored research; informed consent; equitable distribution of burdens and benefits in selecting groups of human subjects; research involving vulnerable persons, children, and women; confidentiality; and disclosure of conflicts of interest. Medical research is limited to what is therapeutic—that is, what may potentially benefit the subject. Application of the guidelines relies on the integrity of the researchers and sponsors.

Complementary Ethical Codes

Large number of physicians and nurses are employed in public health. This means that the codes of ethics of the American Medical Association (AMA) and the American Nurses Association (ANA) are important sources of guidance for these medical professionals, and, consequently, for their work in the organization. Public health managers may be affiliates of the American College of Healthcare Executives (ACHE). Regardless, it is certain that they will interact with health services management professionals who are:

Physicians The first *Principles of Medical Ethics* was adopted by the AMA at its founding in 1847 and was based on the code of medical ethics developed in 1803 by the 19th-century

English physician and philosopher, Sir Thomas Percival (1740–1804) (*Current Opinions of the Judicial Council*, 1982). Subsequent revisions continued to incorporate portions of the Hippocratic philosophy governing physician-patient relationships. The 2001 *Principles* continues the trend of recognizing the profession's responsibilities and the rights of patients that began in 1847. Previous iterations had emphasized benefits and harms as judged by the physician. The *Principles* directs members to "strive to report physicians deficient in character or competence, or engaging in fraud or deception, to appropriate entities." Opinions of the AMA's Council on Ethical and Judicial Affairs assist in interpreting the *Principles*.

Nurses The *Code for Nurses* was first adopted by the ANA in 1950; the latest was adopted in 2001. That iteration has nine provisions, including various expectations: principles to guide practice, primary commitment to the patient, patient advocacy, individual accountability, duties to self and others, improving health care, advancing the profession, collaboration, and obligations to the profession. An interpretive statement follows each. The philosophy of the *Code* is that the goal of nursing is to support the client's responsibility and self-determination to the greatest extent possible. Nurses, too, are expected to act when health care and safety are affected by the incompetent, unethical, or illegal practice of any person.

Health Services Managers The ACHE *Code of Ethics* is reviewed and updated annually; a major revision was adopted in 1987. A primary and contextual focus of the *Code* is protecting and furthering the interests of the patient, client, or others served. Special attention is given to issues such as responsibility to those served by the organization, obligations to the profession and the organization, roles in providing health services to the community and to those in need of services, and conflicts of interest. The *Code* encompasses the concept of *moral agency*, which holds that healthcare executives are morally accountable for the implications of their malfeasance, nonfeasance, and misfeasance. ACHE affiliates are obligated to bring to the attention of the ACHE Ethics Committee any information that reasonably causes them to believe that an affiliate has breached the *Code*.

Summary

Codes of ethics provide an important reference point and context for managers in public health. They are the general context in which the personal ethic resides. The personal ethic may be at variance with professional codes, but this should occur only when there is compelling moral justification. Public health managers should know how and why their personal ethic exceeds the expectations of the professional code and will be hard-pressed to justify performing at a lesser level.

PROFESSIONALISM IN PUBLIC HEALTH

Ethical Issues in Public Health Management

The role of the public health manager in preventing, identifying, and solving ethical problems is multifaceted. The manager's personal ethic has been discussed; its importance would be difficult to overstate. Those without a coherent, comprehensive, and consistent personal ethic will find themselves frustrated and adrift when considering ethical issues and are likely to resort to ethical relativism. As a resource allocator, the public health manager is obligated to provide the support needed by the organization and its staff so that they are educated about ethics issues, have learned a methodology for addressing the ethical dimensions of management and service delivery problems, and have the systems and procedures to support these efforts. Education about the organization's values is an essential first step. In this effort, celebrating heroes of the culture and providing case examples are very useful. In addition, the manager is the driving force in ascertaining that the policies and procedures of the organization address all of the areas where it is likely ethical problems will arise.

Conflicts of Interest

Conflicts of interest are a common and insidious problem in organizations of all types. The healthcare field has not been immune from them, despite the attention devoted to the problem in codes of ethics, professional publications, and the popular press. To paraphrase the poet Carl Sandburg, it is not fog but conflicts of interest that come on little cat feet. Their stealth and insidiousness make them a bane to managers, who must be continually alert lest they become ensnared.

Commonly, they involve personal gain. This is only one of several ways they are evidenced, however. Constant attention and great care in establishing and maintaining relationships will help prevent conflicts of interest from occurring. Even then, however, there is no guarantee that they can be avoided completely. Often, a conflict of interest is also a breach of a fiduciary duty.

Conflicts of interest arise when someone has two sets of duties or obligations (differing interests) and meeting one set makes it impossible to meet the other. These differing interests become a conflict of interest because the decision maker cannot meet the duty of fidelity (loyalty) to both organizations when a decision that affects both is needed. This concept embodies the Biblical admonition against serving two masters. Whether a conflict of interest is present is fact-dependent, and an accurate determination requires careful scrutiny. The potential for a conflict of interest does not necessarily mean that there is a conflict of interest. Even when differing interests are present, it is possible to avoid actual conflicts of interest, but the slope is slippery.

Differing interests are present, for example, when a public health manager has an ownership interest in a vendor that could provide service to the organization. If the manager approves purchases from that vendor at higher-than-market prices, a conflict of interest has occurred. However, if the price is lower than that available elsewhere, the differing interest continues, but no conflict of interests has occurred. In fact, the better pricing is an advantage to the organization. However, if the manager uses the position of authority to cover up inadequacies in the service being provided, the differing interest becomes a conflict of interest.

Some codes of ethics recognize that the line between acceptable and unacceptable behavior is often one of degree. Gifts to decision makers from vendors raise special problems. Pragmatists will argue that the normal conduct of business creates relationships that contain differing interests with the potential for conflicts of interest. It is highly unlikely that making gifts of even modest value has an intention other than to influence managerial decision making in favor of the giver.

Gratuities and Diminished Objectivity

A common source of differing interests occurs when a decision maker in an organization has personal gain from outside relationships. *Gratuities* from vendors are commonly offered to oil the gears of commerce. When gratuities are large or when they are given with the implication that something is expected in return, a differing interest has arisen. Even small gratuities diminish objectivity, and organizations that have guidelines regarding accepting gratuities assist their staffs and express an important cultural value.

Public health practitioners employed by state or local governments are likely to have specific legal requirements regarding conflicts of interest. These include gifts, meals, travel, entertainment, and other types of gratuities beyond a very modest limit. Other inducements are less easily identifiable. An implied reward of employment in the future because of a decision favorable to the vendor now is more subtle and less easily identified. It is unethical, nonetheless.

Even in the presence of statutory or regulatory prohibitions or guidelines, several actions and activities can help public health managers and their organizations avoid conflicts of interest or minimize their effect if they have already occurred. Competitive bidding for procurement of goods and services reduces the likelihood that conflicts of interest will occur, and this is typically required for purchasing by government entities. Education and an awareness of the differing interests that raise the potential for conflicts of interests in all decisions and relationships and consciously seeking to avoid situations where they can occur—prevention—is the most useful approach. Once conflicts have developed, decision makers must disclose them to a higher authority and remove themselves from the decision-making process. In addition, the organization can assist employees who may receive gratuities from sales representatives and drug detailers by developing appropriate policies. A policy that no gratuities can be accepted is the cleanest and clearest approach and leaves nothing to the potential recipient's judgment. Again, as with most aspects of leadership, it is the responsibility of managers at all levels to set an example regarding gratuities.

Managers must avoid even the appearance of a conflict of interest. Few revelations are as devastating to one's moral leadership as the suggestion of improper gain from a position of authority. Managers in the health field are generally held to a higher standard; the mere appearance of impropriety is considered more stringently than the same activity would be if performed in a business enterprise.

Fiduciary Duty

Those in positions of organizational leadership and responsibility are *fiduciaries*. Among the expectations of fiduciaries is that they will avoid conflicts of interest. A fiduciary relationship and its resultant duties are established whenever trust and confidence result in a superior position of influence in another

relationship. Some fiduciary relationships are established by law; for example, someone who is a director of a corporation or who is in a therapeutic relationship, such as a psychiatrist, is a fiduciary, and the law sets high expectations for them. The ethical concept of fiduciary duty is much broader and includes all persons in a position of trust, authority, and responsibility; this includes public health managers. The general ethical and legal guideline is that fiduciaries cannot use their position for personal gain and must act only in the best interests of the entity to whom their duty is owed.

Three examples of breaching a fiduciary duty suggest application of the concept of a fiduciary in public health management: a public health manager who fails to maintain competency in the skills needed to effectively perform, a public health manager whose judgment and effectiveness are impaired because of chemical addiction, and a public health manager so distracted by personal and family problems that job performance is poor.

Consent

Consent is an ethical issue that should concern the public health manager. Several of the codes of ethics discussed earlier give special attention to consent. Operationalizing the autonomy of those served requires that the organization assure itself that there has been adequate, understood, and communicated information as to the services that are to be rendered under its auspices. Consent is obtained after benefits, risks, and alternatives to the services to be rendered have been explained. Organizational policies and procedures should be established to provide assurance that clinical staff ascertain that the person being served adequately understands what is happening. Ethically, managers must recognize the importance of assuring the adequacy of consent, establish the means by which it is accomplished, and provide the staff that will make it a reality.

The legal dimensions of consent in health services are based on the concept that liberty rights prohibit any intervention unless the individual has agreed to it. There are exceptions, such as a presumption of consent in an emergency when a person cannot communicate. Consent can be *implied*, such as going to a public health clinic and asking for treatment, or it can be *express*, as occurs when a consent form is signed after an explanation of risks, benefits, and alternatives to the treatment have been recommended. Three elements are necessary for consent to be ethical:

- *Voluntary.* Consent must be given freely, without coercion or other interference with the decision.
- *Competent.* Consent can only be given by someone who is mentally capable of knowing the nature and consequences of the decision.

- *Informed.* Consent must be based on information that is provided. The usual standard is that the information must be what a reasonable physician would give to a reasonable patient. It includes a discussion of the benefits, risks, and alternatives.

Obtaining consent for clinical decisions that is voluntary, competent, and informed is the legal responsibility of physicians, or someone authorized to act for them. The consent process as undertaken by physicians may be flawed, however. Ethics and the values commonly found in public health organizations strongly suggest that the organization should undertake additional efforts to determine that the patient understands the nature of a treatment or surgical procedure and what is going to happen. Upon inquiry, it may be clear that the patient has agreed to undergo the treatment but does not know what is being done or why. At this point, a process for further education of the patient by the treating physician or a qualified surrogate must be undertaken. Physicians may consider this verification of the adequacy of consent an infringement on their physician–patient relationship. Regardless, it is essential that the consent process is effective. It must be clear to all that what is being sought is a consent process that focuses on the best interests of the patient (beneficence) and mitigates harm (nonmaleficence); all who are involved in it must be advocates for the patient.

Resource Allocation

Resource allocation in public health organizations occurs at the macro and micro level. The macro level includes purchasing capital equipment and implementing or discontinuing a service. These decisions have major resource implications for the organization. In turn, macro allocation has major implications for the micro allocation decisions made by those who provide services. For example, a decision not to offer an education program to promote good oral hygiene in the public schools (macro allocation) will result in more children and young adults visiting the public health dental clinics with caries and impacted teeth (micro allocation). In turn, this increased demand may mean that persons needing other dental services may be unable to obtain them. Macro allocation decisions invariably have direct or indirect health implications, and successful public health managers should involve clinical staff in making them. Nevertheless, resource constraints mean that not all that is desired and desirable in terms of services is available.

Quality of Care

It is estimated that 30% of the cost of providing a good or service results from waste, delay, and rework. In the health services field and in public health, such costs are even more significant because the costs of discomfort, pain, morbidity, and mortality that can occur must be evaluated and added. The public health manager has an ethical obligation to understand the theory of quality improvement and to implement it throughout the organization in all clinical and administrative processes.

An essential first step is to visualize the organization as comprised of large numbers of subsidiary and core processes within the system known as the organization. In this regard, the work of W. Edwards Deming is the most instructive (1986, 2000). Quality can only be improved by making processes more efficient through reengineering, quality improvement, Six Sigma, lean, and similar techniques. Measuring and improving quality is an ethical imperative for managers because doing so will husband resources, diminish morbidity and mortality for persons served, increase staff morale, and generally allow the organization to perform its duties more effectively and efficiently.

Research

The medical field has always engaged in research, which is defined as attempting new means, methods, and techniques. This focus can be found throughout public health. It is obvious that without research, knowledge and progress will stagnate. Protecting the rights and welfare of human subjects is a continuing, important concern, however. To protect human subjects organizations conducting research should establish an institutional review board (IRB), which is an independent committee comprised of scientific and nonscientific members that meets the requirements of federal law (*Code of Federal Regulations* [CFR], Title 45, Part 46 & Title 21, Part 56). It is almost certain that state law will require government organizations to establish IRBs that will conduct initial and continued review of research involving human subjects. Committees with similar activities are also considered IRBs.

The Department of Health and Human Services (HHS) and the Food and Drug Administration (FDA) are the most important federal entities that require an IRB to review, approve, and maintain oversight of research studies. HHS requirements for IRBs and protection of human subjects are applicable to research funded [i.e., supported (or conducted by) and regulated under a specific research statute] by 17 federal agencies and departments that have adopted the "common rule" or "federal policy" for the protection of human subjects (Barnes & Krauss, 2000).

Research involving human subjects that is funded wholly or partly by the federal government must be reviewed by an IRB with a process that meets HHS criteria. Although technically not required, research funding applications typically include assurances that the organization will comply with HHS IRB requirements for human subjects (and other HHS requirements for the protection of human subjects) for *all* its research, whether or not federally funded (Barnes & Krauss, 2000). The FDA regulates interstate sale of drugs, biologicals, and medical devices and has the same requirements as HHS. The FDA regulates neither surgical experimentation nor innovative clinical care, which is defined as *new* uses of existing treatments, drugs, biologicals (i.e., vaccines), and devices.

Membership and Purpose

Institutions may choose specific IRB members, but federal regulations (and perhaps state law) govern composition of membership, nature of the review conducted, and conflicts of interest of IRB members (Barnes & Krauss, 2000). IRBs review research proposals for conformance with the law, standards of professional conduct and practice, and institutional commitment and regulations. IRBs acceptable to HHS have a minimum of five members with varying backgrounds (at least one must have professional interests that are scientific and one whose interests are nonscientific) and who are capable of reviewing research proposals and activities of the type commonly performed by the organization (45 CFR 46.107).

IRBs acceptable to HHS must apply specific requirements when reviewing research activities (45 CFR 46.111):

- Risks to subjects are minimized.
- Risks to subjects are reasonable in relation to anticipated benefit, if any.
- Selection of research subjects is equitable.
- Informed consent is sought from each prospective subject or the subject's legally authorized representative.
- Informed consent is appropriately documented.
- When appropriate, the research plan has adequate provision for monitoring the data collected to ensure the safety of subjects.
- When appropriate, there are adequate provisions to protect the privacy of subjects and maintain the confidentiality of data.

Additional safeguards are required when some or all of the subjects are likely to be vulnerable to coercion or undue influence; examples include children, prisoners, pregnant women, mentally disabled persons, or the economically or educationally disadvantaged. Several provisions identify the information needed for informed consent.

Requirements Regulations issued in 1981 eliminated the requirement that any HHS funding to an organization *required* use of HHS guidelines in *all* research, regardless of funding source. This change increased the importance of the role of managers and researchers and put greater reliance on the organization's policies and procedures and on managers' personal ethic.

As a practical matter, organizations with multiple research funding sources, one of them federal, are likely to use the same HHS-qualified IRB for all research protocols. It is easy to slip, however, and managers must be alert to potential ethical problems in formal research programs, as well as in isolated innovative therapy or surgical experimentation.

It has been forcefully argued that nondiagnostic and nontherapeutic (no therapeutic benefit to the subject) research on children and adults who are legally incompetent should be prohibited (Ramsey, 1970). Nontherapeutic research on children is permitted, however. A risk-benefit ratio is applied, and no child can be placed in unnecessary jeopardy. Assent from the child and consent from parents or legally authorized representatives are required. The ethical, economic, political, legal, and scientific problems of research involving children are daunting, however, and researchers are reluctant to undertake it. Congress *has not* given the FDA authority to *require* extensive testing on children. Despite efforts by Congress and the FDA to encourage testing of pharmaceuticals and biologicals on children, little research involving them is done, and most prescribing for children is based on physician trial and error (Budetti, 2003). It is estimated that 50% to 75% of drugs used in pediatric medicine have not been studied adequately to provide appropriate labeling information (Roberts, Rodriguez, Murphy, & Crescenzi, 2003).

Exempt Research and Research Warranting Expedited Review
Six categories of research are exempt from HHS requirements. Examples are research conducted in established or normally accepted educational settings involving normal educational practices; research involving use of educational tests, survey and interview procedures, or observation of public behavior; and research involving the collection or study of existing data, documents, records, and pathological or diagnostic specimens. Limits are specified (Summary of Basic Protections, 1997).

HHS regulations identify research warranting expedited review as a category to which different provisions apply. Expedited review allows special procedures for approval of certain types of research that pose no more than minimal risk to human subjects (45 CFR 46.110). Examples of research categories appropriate to expedited review are clinical studies of drugs and medical devices, collection of blood samples, collection of biological specimens such as hair and nail clippings and deciduous teeth, and collection of data through noninvasive procedures (Categories of Research, 1998). Expedited review greatly facilitates several kinds of research.

Summary Regulations such as those imposed by HHS focus responsibility on the organization and its IRB. Regardless of legal requirements, public health managers have independent ethical duties to protect research subjects under the principles of respect for persons, beneficence, nonmaleficence, and even justice (e.g., fairly allocating support for research). The virtues of honesty, integrity, and trustworthiness are also applicable. Managers must establish and maintain systems and procedures to prevent unauthorized research and to provide the necessary extra protection when innovative treatment or surgical research is proposed or undertaken. Most important are staff awareness about the parameters of acceptable practice and the courage to act. Despite all of the supposed safeguards—especially in governmental facilities—human subjects continue to be at considerable risk (Hudson, 2008).

Cultural and Spiritual Diversity

The past several decades have witnessed enhanced attention to cultural and spiritual diversity. These changes have resulted from a greater sensitivity to the presence of various ethnic and cultural groups in the United States. Some of this attention is reflected in federal law, such as that creating the Equal Employment Opportunity Commission and similar laws in various states. Such laws provide a legal framework in which employment and other relationships (as well as their "ethic") are judged. These and similar laws also created protected classes. Thus, unlawful discrimination, accommodating diversity, sexual harassment, intimate or romantic relationships in the workplace, sexual orientation, affirmative action, and diversity programs all raise ethical (and oftentimes legal) issues that the organization must address if it is to act ethically.

Public health organizations and their managers must obey the law as a minimum level of performance. In addition, however, they are expected to be especially aware of the special needs of groups and individuals, whether the relationships are one of service, employment, or in the general conduct of service delivery. It is important to stress that there is no expectation that the organization's legally compliant value system as expressed in its statement of organizational philosophy or other guiding principles must be breached to meet the demands of patients, clients, or others served, or of employees. This position is generally accepted by the courts for private (nongovernmental) corporations, but governmental facilities may not enforce theologically based positions because this has been interpreted by the courts as constituting an unconstitutional establishment of religion. Thus, governmental facilities provide services that nongovernmental facilities may not be forced to provide.

Cultural sensitivity and awareness are especially important for organizations attempting to deliver services to diverse populations. For example, various cultures and religions have widely differing views of illness, dying, and death. These views determine the roles and reactions not only of the patient but of family and friends, as well as what is seen as the appropriate role of the organization and providers. Organizations that have ethnically and culturally diverse staff can draw on them as resources in such situations. Public health organizations should accommodate the religious and social beliefs and customs of persons served when possible, but only to the extent that the organization's mission is not compromised and other persons being served are not put at risk or have their services jeopardized.

Educating Public Health Practitioners

The education of public health practitioners raises several ethical issues. Foremost among them is to consent to be treated by someone in training. Clinical and field experience are required as part of the training for most types of public health practitioners. Students in medicine, public health nursing, biostatistics, epidemiology, and management benefit greatly by having a period of training at the type of organization in which they will do their professional work. Those in training roles must be clearly identified, and their status must be known to all with whom they have contact. This information is especially important when those in training are interacting with persons served. In addition, persons who receive services may be expressly or implicitly misled as to the training of those involved. This is a perversion of utilitarian thinking—the ends of education justify the means of misleading those served. The principle of respect for persons—specifically, truth telling—demands that persons be informed of the identities and roles of their caregivers.

Politicization of Public Health

A discussion of ethics in public health would be incomplete without recognizing the significant risk of organizational or programmatic politicization. Public health organizations and public health practitioners have a unique relationship to government and the political process. They are largely dependent on the goodwill of government and politicians for their continued existence. As with any publicly funded entity, the risk is great that they will fall prey to prevailing political viewpoints and become caught up in political correctness to the exclusion of objective decision making. Such problems are most likely to arise in macro resource allocation. If public health organizations and practitioners lose, or appear to lose, their scientific objectivity because they are too closely tied to one political point of view, the public will lose confidence in them—they will be seen as merely an extension of a political point of view. As noted earlier, trust, once lost, is very hard to regain. It takes courage and the ability to persuade through the use of science and objectively defensible data to protect the public's health without diminishing their autonomy or violating the precepts of beneficence, nonmaleficence, and justice for all in the public. Successful managers must have a well-developed, clearly identifiable personal ethic.

Preventing and Solving Ethical Problems

Ethics committees are common in health care, and they should be considered for public health organizations. Ethics committees could provide consultation for ethics issues that arise in clinical programs; serve as a repository of expertise and case-based experience (as suggested by the discussion on casuistry); educate staff; and prospectively consider the ethical implications of policies, procedures, and resource allocation. In addition, the ethics committee could be involved in preventing and resolving management ethics problems such as conflicts of in-

terest. Support for an ethics committee by management should include a small budget, modest staff assistance, and the prestige of recognizing their importance in the organization. Ethicists may be used as consultants to aid the process at minimal cost.

CONCLUSION

The most important message of this chapter is that each of us is a moral agent. Our actions and inactions have moral implications for us and for all who are affected by them. Each of us must have a well-considered, comprehensive personal ethic that is the lodestar in our professional and personal lives, which, as noted earlier, merge in many ways as public health managers. We will be most effective as managers if we lead by example and are a model of ethical behavior.

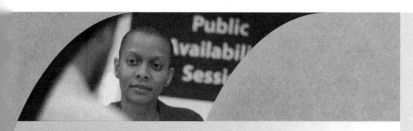

Discussion Questions

1. What is the connection of law to ethics? Provide examples of the dynamics of that relationship, especially as to how one affects and is affected by the other.

2. Identify sources that contribute to a personal ethic. Explain why a personal ethic evolves over time.

3. What is the relationship between a manager's personal ethic and the organization's philosophy and values? How does the manager positively (and negatively) affect the organization's values and culture?

4. How do utilitarianism and Kantian deontology vie for ascendency in public health decision making?

5. How should the four ethical principles be applied in an operational setting? Should they be found in policies, procedures, and rules that affect decision making in the organization? Why or why not?

6. How do managers identify and avoid conflicts of interest? What is the role of the organization in terms of conflicts of interest?

7. Identify the risks of politicization of resource allocation in public health. Provide examples of how public health decisions can diminish personal liberty.

REFERENCES

American Medical Association. *Current Opinions of the Judicial Council, vii.* Chicago: American Medical Association; 1982.

Arras J, Rhoden N. *Ethical Issues in Modern Medicine.* 3rd ed. Mountain View, CA: Mayfield Publishing; 1989.

Barnes M, Krauss S. Conflicts of interest in human research: risks and pitfalls of 'easy money' in research funding. *BNA's Health Law Reporter.* August 2000;9(35):1382-1383.

Beauchamp T, Walters L. *Contemporary Issues in Bioethics.* 4th ed. Belmont, CA: Wadsworth; 1994:21.

Bodenheimer E. *Jurisprudence: The Philosophy and Method of the Law.* Revised ed. Cambridge, MA: Harvard University Press; 1962.

Budetti PB. Ensuring safe and effective medications for children. *JAMA.* 2003;290(7):950-951.

Carney F. Theological Ethics. In: Reich W, ed. *Encyclopedia of Bioethics.* Vol 1. New York: The Free Press; 1978:435-436.

Darr K. Adapted from Chapter 1. *Ethics in Health Services Management.* 4th ed. Baltimore: Health Professions Press; 2005.

Deming WE. *Out of the Crisis.* Boston: MIT; 1986:18.

Deming WE. *The New Economics for Industry, Government, Education.* 2nd ed. Cambridge, MA: MIT-CAES; 2000.

Henderson VE. The ethical side of enterprise. *Sloan Management Review.* 1982;23:41-42. Can a corporation know the difference between right and wrong? In *State v. Christy-Pontiac, GMC, Inc.* (354 N.W.2d 17), the Minnesota Supreme Court held that a corporation could form the specific intent necessary to commit theft and forgery and thus be subject to criminal fines. The irony of the case lies in the fact that corporate officers were found not guilty when tried separately on the same charges (Simonett, John E. "A Corporation's Soul." *Minnesota Bench & Bar,* September (1997): 34–35.

Hudson A. Violations rife in hospital's studies on veterans: Inspector general finds consent forms, death reports missing. *The Washington Times.* August 5, 2008:A1.

Jonsen A. Casuistry and Clinical Ethics. *Theoretical Medicine.* 1986;7:71.

Jonsen A, Toulmin S. *The Abuse of Casuistry: A History of Moral Reasoning.* Berkeley: University of California Press; 1988:13.

Kant I. Fundmental Principles of the Metaphysics of Morals. In: Sprague E, Taylor PW, eds. Abbott TK, trans. *Knowledge and Value.* New York: Harcourt, Brace; 1959:535-558.

Nelson WA, Weeks WB, Campfield JM. The organizational costs of ethical conflicts. *Journal of Healthcare Management* 53, no. 1 (January–February 2008): 41–53.

Pellegrino ED, Thomasma DC. *For the Patient's Good: The Restoration of Beneficence in Health Care.* New York: Oxford University Press; 1988.

Pellegrino ED. The Virtuous Physician and the Ethics of Medicine. In Beauchamp TL, Walters L, eds. *Comtemporary Issues in Bioethics,* 4th ed. Belmont, CA: Wadsworth Publishing, 1994.

"Principles of the Ethical Practice of Public Health, Version 2.2." Public Health Leadership Society, 2002.

Ramsey P. Research involving children or incompetents. *The Patient as Person.* New Haven, CT: Yale University Press; 1970:252.

Rawls J. *A Theory of Justice.* Cambridge, MA: Belknap Press; 1971:60.

Roberts R, Rodriguez W, Murphy D, Crescenzi T. Pediatric drug labeling: Improving the safety and efficacy of pediatric therapies. *JAMA.* 2003;290(7):905-911.

Society for Public Health Education. *Ethics.* 2003. http://www.sophe.org/ethics.cfm. Accessed July 23, 2008.

Summary of Basic Protections for Human Subjects. (1997, December 23). Office for Protection from Research Risks. http://ohrp.osophs.dhhs.gov/humansubjects/guidance/basics.htm, retrieved August 17, 2003.

U.S. Code of Federal Regulations (CFR). Title 45, Part 46, and Title 21, Part 56.

United States Department of Health and Human Services. *45 CFR 46.107, IRB Membership, effective July 14, 2009.* http://www.hhs.gov/ohrp/humansubjects/guidance/45cfr46.htm#46.107.

United States Department of Health and Human Services. *45 CRF 46.110, Expedited Review Procedures for Certain Kinds of Research Involving No More Than Minimal Risk, and for Minor Changes in Approved Research, effective July 14, 2009.* http://www.hhs.gov/ohrp/humansubjects/guidance/45cfr46.htm#46.110.

United States Department of Health and Human Services. *45 CFR 46.111, Criteria for IRB Approval of Research, effective July 14, 2009.* http://www.hhs.gov/ohrp/humansubjects/guidance/45cfr46.htm#46.111.

United States Department of Health and Human Services. *Categories of Research that May Be Reviewed by the Institutional Review Board (IRB) through an Expedited Review.* http://www.hhs.gov/ohrp/requests/com102607.html.

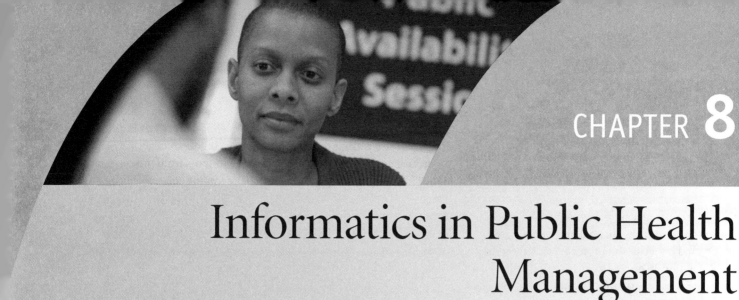

CHAPTER **8**

Informatics in Public Health Management

Philip Aspden

INTRODUCTION

Perhaps there is no greater example of the dramatic change in our daily lives than the changes in the availability of electronic devices, the information these devices provide, and the systems that support these devices. Personal computers, mobile phones, global positioning systems (to name just a few examples) that were few and far between even 10 years ago, are now commonplace, even in the most remote places on earth. The increasing functionality and ever-lower prices of these devices bring the ability to collect and analyze data more cheaply than ever before and the need for systematic approaches by the organizations that deploy and operate these devices.

For the first time in our history, public health data are readily and relatively cheaply available. These data, their interpretation, and the strategic and operational plans that can be derived from these data are the very foundation of good public health as well as public health management, policy, and regulation. It is the responsibility of the well-trained public health manager and leader to be comfortable in this rapidly expanding area of public health informatics. Simply stated, *public health informatics* is the systematic application of information technology to public health practice, research, and learning (O'Carroll, 2003). Public health informatics is distinguished by:

- A focus on population health data rather than on individual health data.
- Large (multimillion) record databases able to efficiently carry out analyses such as cross-tabulations and trending.
- The reuse of data originally collected for other (usually treatment) purposes—hence, networks for collecting data are an important part of public health informatics.

- Systems being established and operated, either directly or indirectly, by federal, state, or city governments.

This chapter focuses on five key public health information system applications: reporting systems, registries, surveys, electronic knowledge sources, and networks for linking public health professionals. The different data types used in these applications, the functionality provided by these applications, and the information technology issues relating to using and implementing the applications are discussed as well. The public health manager needs to be cognizant of the more common data sources and systems to be able to manage public health agencies effectively. Those who are interested in learning more details about the applications and systems should review the references at the end of the chapter or visit the suggested Web sites.

1. *Reporting systems.* Public health surveillance is the routine and systematic collection, analysis, interpretation, and reporting of population-based data for the purposes of detecting, characterizing, and countering threats to public health. Traditional systems utilize voluntary reporting, initially through paper-based reports sent by mail, and later, through reports sent via computer networks. More recently, surveillance systems have been developed that automatically acquire data daily or more frequently. These near-real-time systems offer the promise of earlier detection of threats to public health.

2. *Registries.* Disease registries are regional, national, or sometimes multinational databases that collect longitudinal clinical data on patients with a particular disease

(e.g., breast cancer). The analysis of the data is used to develop and test hypotheses about the etiology, transmission, and risk factors that contribute to the particular disease. Immunization registries are another type of public health registry. These registries are population-based, computerized information systems that collect vaccination data about population groups, particularly children. They are used by patients, parents, providers, and public health professionals to keep track of vaccination histories to ensure that children and other groups receive timely immunizations.

3. *Surveys*. Periodic surveys are useful for augmenting the reporting systems and for providing information in public health areas where reporting systems are lacking. Some surveys consist of information collected during a personal interview, augmented by collection of clinical information. Surveys should also provide a more representative sample of population health than the results of voluntary reporting systems. In many cases, the survey data are made available for public health specialists to analyze for themselves.

4. *Electronic knowledge sources*. Reporting systems, registries, and surveys provide qualitative and quantitative data about a particular population at a given time. Such data can be analyzed to produce knowledge or insights into the variability of the data and relationships between the data elements. With the emergence of the Internet, much knowledge is now available electronically. For the public health professional, three types of electronic knowledge source are of importance: bibliographic databases (e.g., MEDLINE), subject matter databases (e.g., Hazardous Substance Data Bank), and databases of systematic reviews (e.g., the Cochrane Collaboration).

5. *Networks for linking public health professionals and responding to public health emergencies*. Sharing information about public health events among public health officials is often crucial to identifying serious threats to public health. Networks exist at the federal (e.g., CDC's Epi-X) and state (e.g., Florida's EpiCom) levels for public health officials for sharing postings and discussions about disease outbreaks and other public health events that potentially involve multiple jurisdictions. Networks are also important for responding to public health emergencies.

The material given in this chapter describes various systems and networks that help the public health professional and manager learn about threats to the public's health and devise ways to protect or improve the nation's health. Public health managers and leaders are responsible, either directly or indirectly, for ensuring that the various stakeholders[1] are aware of the benefits of such systems, that the outputs from these systems are effectively used, that these systems are correctly budgeted, and that new developments that meet the needs of the public health community are implemented.

LEARNING OBJECTIVES

After reading this chapter, the reader will be able to:

1. Describe the functionality of the main public health information system applications.
2. Identify the information technology skill sets needed to effectively use these applications.
3. Describe the development, implementation, and management of public health information technology systems.
4. Identify background on key public health information applications (such as morbidity reporting, automated surveillance systems, disease and immunization registries, morbidity and risk factor surveys, electronic knowledge sources, and telecommunications networks for linking public health professionals).
5. Identify the details of the information technology skills needed to effectively use these applications (searching and analyzing databases, public health data standards, and building and managing information systems).

PUBLIC HEALTH INFORMATION SYSTEM APPLICATIONS

Reporting Systems

The National Center for Health Statistics (NCHS) at the Centers for Disease Control and Prevention (CDC) is the principal health statistics agency in the United States for collecting data to aid healthcare policy development and implementation (NCHS, 2008a). It develops and maintains both reporting systems that collect vital statistics data and carries out surveys (discussed later) that collect national morbidity and health risk assessment data. Another part of the CDC, the Division of Surveillance and Epidemiology (DSE), is responsible for the national compilation of notifiable diseases reported weekly by state and territorial epidemiologists. A number of federal and state patient safety reporting systems have been established that seek ways to deliver safer health care following analyses of reported cases. Accessing and using the data are discussed in a later section of this chapter.

Stakeholder refers to the constellation of all who are involved in public health. The stakeholders include clinicians, government officials, providers, and, most importantly, the citizens themselves.

Vital Statistics Data

The national vital statistics system that collects data on births, deaths, and marriages is a collaborative effort between state and federal agencies. States collect the data and the National Center for Health Statistics combines the state-collected data to create a national database. To ensure the uniformity needed to combine the data sets from each state, the NCHS recommends standards for states to adopt for data collection. Originally, the data collection was completely paper-based, but gradually the process has become automated.

Since 1996, the NCHS has released vital statistics data on CD-ROM (Freedman and Weed, 2003) and more recently via the Web. Key data sets of interest to public health professionals are births, deaths, fetal deaths, linked birth/infant deaths, and perinatal deaths. Each record includes demographic and health information derived from the birth or death certificate, as appropriate.

Morbidity Reporting

Public health surveillance is the reporting of infectious diseases and conditions of public health interest. State and territory public health officials and the CDC jointly determine which diseases and conditions should be under national surveillance (Roush et al., 1999). The list is available from the CDC website (http://www.cdc.gov/ncphi/disss/nndss/PHS/infdis2008.htm), although the list of what is reported by each state and territory varies. Originally, nurses and doctors were the primary source of disease reporting, but recently laboratories have also become important sources of reporting. In some places, especially in rural areas, trained community healthcare workers who are paraprofessionals are reliable sources of health data (Institute of Medicine [IOM], 2007). The CDC publishes weekly and annual summaries of the data submitted by states and territories.

Prior to 2000, state health departments received most notifiable disease reports by mail and then entered the data into computer systems, often weeks after the cases had occurred. In addition, there was significant underreporting, and more than 100 different systems were used to transmit these reports from the states to the CDC (Morbidity and Mortality Weekly Report [MMWR], 2005). To improve the quantity and timeliness of reporting, the CDC established the National Electronic Disease Surveillance System (NEDSS), an initiative that promotes the use of data and information system standards to foster the development of integrated and interoperable surveillance systems at federal, state, and local levels (http://www.cdc.gov/NEDSS). NEDSS is a major component of the Public Health Information Network (PHIN), which is discussed later. In

September 2000, states began receiving federal funding to plan and implement NEDSS-compatible systems (MMWR, 2005). Sixteen states (including Tennessee, Texas, and Vermont) (*Federal Register*, 2007), as of late 2007, have implemented the NEDSS Base System, a comprehensive reporting system developed by the CDC, while other states (e.g., Pennsylvania) (Pennsylvania Department of Health [PA-DOH], 2008) have developed their own systems based on NEDSS standards.

Patient Safety Reporting Systems

The federal government operates several patient safety reporting systems—for example, the National Nosocomial Infections Surveillance (NNIS) System, the Dialysis Surveillance Network, the Adverse Event Reporting System, and the Vaccine Adverse Event Reporting System. The aim of all these systems is to collect data on adverse events and then to analyze these data to identify ways to improve the safety of the delivery of health care.

The Adverse Event Reporting System (AERS) is a computerized information database designed to support the U.S. Food and Drug Administration's (FDA) post-marketing safety surveillance program for all approved drug and therapeutic biologic products. Serious adverse events and product problems are reported directly to the FDA or via the manufacturer. Reports are sent in by mail or fax or via a Web interface. Reporting requirements vary: reporting is voluntary for consumers and health professionals but mandatory for healthcare facilities such as hospitals. On a quarterly basis, subsets of the data included in all the received reports are made available to public health researchers and others.

The Institute of Medicine report, *To Err Is Human* (IOM, 2000), raised significant concerns about healthcare quality problems. These concerns led to the establishment of state patient safety reporting systems. As of October 2007, 26 states plus the District of Columbia had passed legislation or introduced regulations related to hospital reporting of adverse events to a state agency (National Academy for State Health Policy [NASHP], 2008). For example in Pennsylvania, state legislation requires Pennsylvania-licensed hospitals, birthing centers, ambulatory surgical facilities, and selected abortion facilities to report adverse events and near misses to the Pennsylvania Patient Safety Authority using the Pennsylvania Patient Safety Reporting System (PA-PSRS).

Many of the reporting requirements are intended to hold healthcare facilities accountable for weaknesses in their systems. They also have the potential to improve patient safety through event report analysis and by dissemination of best practices and lessons learned that could prevent recurrences. For example, PA-PSRS provides advisory articles throughout the year via its website (PA-PSRS, 2008).

Automated Surveillance Systems

Traditional morbidity reporting systems rely on voluntary reporting, which usually leads to significant underreporting. (MMWR, 2005). Automated systems capture data (e.g., data collected from outpatient visits, or laboratories) periodically throughout the day. These near real-time systems hold the promise of speedier and more comprehensive reporting. Information from outpatient encounters such as diagnosis (using ICD codes) or chief complaint is mapped onto syndromes with software tools identifying unusually high daily syndrome counts. Initially these systems were directed at identifying bioterrorist attacks, but the technology has also been used for general public health applications. Automated surveillance systems have been implemented at federal, state, and city levels:

- BioSense is a near-real-time national surveillance system developed by the CDC. It draws data from Department of Defense and Department of Veteran Affairs treatment facilities and national laboratories (Bradley et al., 2005). The future plans for BioSense include analyzing relevant over-the-counter drug sales and poison control data (CDC, 2008).
- The New Jersey Communicable Disease Reporting and Surveillance System is used to collect electronic laboratory reports of Lyme disease (McHugh et al., 2008). Using the system, the total number of Lyme disease reports increased fivefold, while the number of confirmed reports increased only 18 percent.
- The New York City Department of Health and Mental Hygiene has established an electronic syndrome surveillance system that monitors chief complaint information relating to emergency department visits (Heffernan et al., 2004). Respiratory, fever, diarrhea, and vomiting are the key syndromes analyzed.

Registries

Public health registries are computer applications used to capture, store, and analyze information on persons who have a particular disease, a condition, or exposure to hazardous situations that predisposes to the occurrence of adverse health events, or who have received a healthcare intervention (e.g., an immunization). The information contained in the registry is obtained from multiple sources on a periodic basis and entered into the registry either manually or electronically. The information on a particular individual in a public health registry will only be a fraction of the information contained in the individual's electronic health record. A registry consists of a database to store the information on individuals and software applications for viewing and analyzing the data and providing reports.

Depending on the type of data collected, there are many public health uses of registry data, including:

- Analysis of disease incidence rates to estimate the magnitude of the problem, estimate trends in disease incidence, and identify risk factors and groups particularly at risk.
- Analysis of the treatments received to monitor the adoption of recommended treatments and to identify variations (e.g., across regions) in the delivery of recommended treatments (disease registries).
- Analysis of patient outcomes to estimate survivorship, to compare treatments (generally), and for particular demographic groupings.
- Analysis of the immunization status of a provider's patient (to enable the provider to send out reminders) or of the whole community/high-risk groups within the community (to enable the public health community to target advertising campaigns) (immunization registries).

Registries are operated by a wide range of organizations including the federal government, state governments, universities, hospital groups, and nonprofit organizations, including:

- The National Exposure Registry (www.atsdr.cdc.gov/ner/index.html), operated by the Agency for Toxic Substances and Disease Registry, CDC, monitors the health of those exposed to hazardous substances.
- The U.S. Eye Injury Registry (http://www.useironline.org/index2.html), sponsored by the Helen Keller Eye Research Foundation, provides epidemiologic data that assist with the development of eye injury prevention and management strategies.
- The Wisconsin Immunization Registry, established by state statute and managed by the Wisconsin Department of Health and Family Services, tracks immunizations given to children and adults in the state (Heitz, 2005).

Surveys

Surveys are useful for augmenting the findings of reporting/surveillance systems by providing information on the overall morbidity and unhealthy behaviors of particular demographic groups. The data collected by the surveys are used by the public health research community for epidemiologic and policy analysis, such as characterizing those with various health problems, determining barriers to accessing and using appropriate health care, and evaluating federal health programs. Again, accessing and using survey data is considered later in this chapter.

Morbidity Data

The major morbidity surveys carried out by the NCHS are as follows:

- The National Health Interview Survey (NHIS) is the principal source of information on the health of the civilian noninstitutionalized population of the United States. The National Health Survey Act of 1956 provided for a continuing survey and special studies to secure accurate and current statistical information on the amount, distribution, and effects of illness and disability in the United States and the services rendered for or because of such conditions.
- The National Health and Nutrition Examination Survey (NHANES) is a program of studies designed to assess the health and nutritional status of adults and children in the United States. This survey is particularly important in that it combines interviews and physical examinations. The NHANES interview includes demographic, socioeconomic, dietary, and health-related questions. The physical examination component consists of medical, dental, and physiological measurements, as well as laboratory tests administered by medical personnel. All participants visit a physician. Dietary interviews and body measurements are also included. All but the very young have a blood sample taken and undergo a dental screening.
- National Health Care Surveys address factors that influence the use of healthcare resources; the quality of health care, including safety; and disparities in healthcare services provided to population subgroups in the United States in ambulatory, hospital, and long-term care settings. The surveys include:
  - National Ambulatory Medical Care Survey (NAMCS)
  - National Hospital Ambulatory Medical Care Survey (NHAMCS)
  - National Hospital Discharge Survey (NHDS)
  - National Survey of Ambulatory Surgery (NSAS)
  - National Home and Hospice Care Survey (NHHCS)
  - National Nursing Home Survey (NNHS)
- The National Immunization Survey (NIS) is a survey of those responsible for the immunization of children aged 19 to 35 months and is used to produce estimates of vaccination coverage rates for all childhood vaccinations recommended by the Advisory Committee on Immunization Practices (ACIP).
- The State and Local Area Integrated Telephone Survey (SLAITS) provides a mechanism to collect data quickly on a broad range of topics at the national, state, and local levels. A partial list of examples of research areas

include health insurance coverage, access to care, perceived health status, utilization of services, and measurement of child well-being.

Risk Factor Data

Surveys of risky or unhealthy behavior are carried out by National Center for Health Statistics and the National Center for Chronic Disease Prevention and Health Promotion (NCCDPHP), both part of the CDC. These surveys include:

- The National Mortality Followback Survey, carried out by the NCHS, uses a sample of U.S. residents who die in a given year to supplement the information contained in the death certificate with information from the next of kin or another person familiar with the decedent's life history. This information, sometimes enhanced by administrative records, provides an opportunity to study the etiology of disease, demographic trends in mortality, and other health issues.
- The Youth Risk Behavior Surveillance System (YRBSS), carried out by the NCCDPHP, monitors important health-risk behaviors and the prevalence of obesity and asthma among youth and young adults. The YRBSS includes a national school-based survey conducted by the CDC and state, territorial, tribal, and local surveys conducted by state, territorial, and local education and health agencies and tribal governments.
- Behavior Risk Factor Surveillance Survey (BRFSS), carried out by the NCCDPHP, is a state-based system of health surveys that collects information on health risk behaviors, preventive health practices, and healthcare access primarily related to chronic disease and injury. For many states, the BRFSS is the only available source of timely, accurate data on health-related behaviors.

Electronic Knowledge Sources

Hersh (1996) identified three levels of knowledge bases: primary—original research reports in journals (e.g., the *American Journal of Public Health*), books, and proceedings; secondary—knowledge bases that compile or utilize primary sources to produce bibliographic or factual databases; and tertiary—sources that provide reviews or syntheses of the primary literature. This section focuses on secondary and tertiary sources.

Secondary Knowledge Bases: Bibliographic

Bibliographic databases provide information on journal articles, books, and proceedings, such as the authors' names and affiliations, article title, citation, an abstract or summary of the article/document, and lists of the key topics covered. Sometimes electronic links to the text are provided. Examples of bibliographic databases of relevance to public health professionals include:

- MEDLINE via PubMed (http://www.ncbi.nlm.nih.gov/pubmed/), compiled by the National Library of Medicine (NLM), is a source of life sciences and biomedical bibliographic information, containing nearly 11 million records from more than 7,000 different publications.
- TOXLINE via TOXNET (http://toxnet.nlm.nih.gov/), also compiled by NLM, is a source of references to literature on biochemical, pharmacological, physiological, and toxicological effects of drugs and other chemicals.
- PsycINFO (http://www.apa.org/psycinfo/), compiled by the American Psychological Association, is an abstract database of psychological literature.
- CINAHL (http://www.cinahl.com/library/library.htm), complied by EBSCO Industries, is a database that covers the nursing and allied health literature.
- CDC Wonder (http://wonder.cdc.gov) provides access to CDC reports and public health data.

Secondary Knowledge Bases: Factual

The NLM Specialized Information Service's Toxicology and Environmental Health Information Program (http://tox.nlm.nih.gov) produces TOXNET (http://toxnet.nlm.nih.gov), a collection of toxicology and environmental health databases. TOXNET includes:

- Hazardous Substances Data Bank (HSDB) (http://toxnet.nlm.nih.gov/cgi-bin/sis/htmlgen?HSDB), a database of potentially hazardous chemicals.
- TOXLINE (http://toxnet.nlm.nih.gov/cgi-bin/sis/htmlgen?TOXLINE), mentioned previously.
- ChemIDplus (http://toxnet.nlm.nih.gov/cgi-bin/sis/htmlgen?CHEM), a chemical dictionary and structure database.
- TOXMAP (http://toxmap.nlm.nih.gov/), a resource that uses maps of the United States to show the amount and location of certain toxic chemicals released into the environment.
- WISER (http://wiser.nlm.nih.gov) is a system designed to assist first responders in hazardous material incidents.
- Haz-Map (http://hazmap.nlm.nih.gov) links jobs and hazardous tasks with occupational diseases and their symptoms.
- DIRLINE (http://dirline.nlm.nih.gov/), a directory of organizations and other resources in health and biomedicine.

Tertiary Knowledge Bases

A tertiary knowledge base consists of systematic reviews of the effectiveness of healthcare prevention strategies/treatments by panels of experts looking at the quality of both the experimental design and the analysis of the experimental data and assessing the relative contributions of the relevant research. Two key tertiary knowledge bases are:

- National Guideline Clearinghouse (http://www.guideline.gov), a public resource for evidence-based clinical practice guidelines—an initiative of the Agency for Healthcare Research and Quality.
- The Cochrane Collaboration (http://www.cochrane.org) provides systematic reviews of the effects of healthcare interventions and prevention strategies.

Networks for Linking Public Health Professionals

Speedy communications among public health professionals is key to identifying and responding to public health threats. The CDC has developed an overarching network infrastructure that embraces a number of application-specific networks (e.g., NEDSS). In addition to the federal networks, there are many state-level network initiatives.

Federal Networks

The Public Health Information Network (PHIN) is the CDC's overarching nationwide business and technical architecture for public health information systems (Loonsk et al., 2006). The PHIN was first funded in 2004 to help advance and coordinate public health information systems. Substantial work has gone into developing industry standard specifications for data exchange messages, terminologies, and technologies (Loonsk et al., 2006), including the following:

- Industry standard messaging specifications: Health Level 7 (HL7) implementation guides for disease case reports, laboratory tests, and laboratory results, and for the exchange of certain clinical care data with public health.
- Industry standard terminologies for messages and data models: Logical Observation Identifier Names and Codes (LOINC), Systematized Nomenclature of Medicine (SNOMED), ICD-10 for mortality, and ICD-9CM for morbidity.
- Strong security and secure exchange of data over the Internet using e-Gov technical architecture standards and public key infrastructure (PKI).
- Directories of public health and clinical personnel used to identify people, roles, and contact information for public health participants.

- Alerts and notifications for public health and clinical personnel use.

The various messaging and terminology standards mentioned are discussed in more detail in the public health data standards section.

As mentioned earlier, the PHIN embraces a number of application-specific networks such as NEDSS and the following networks that were developed prior to the establishment of the PHIN:

- The CDC's Epidemic Information Exchange (Epi-X) (http://www.cdc.gov/mmwr/epix/epix.html) is a secure, Web-based communications network that serves as a communications exchange among CDC, state, and local health departments; poison control centers; and other public health professionals. The system provides rapid reporting, immediate notification, and coordination of health investigations for public health professionals. Participation in Epi-X is limited to public health officials designated by health agencies.
- The CDC's Health Alert Network (HAN) (http://www2a.cdc.gov/han/Index.asp) is a nationwide program to establish the communications, distance-learning, and organizational infrastructure to identify and respond to health threats, including the possibility of bioterrorism. It enables local, state, and federal health authorities to communicate and coordinate rapidly and securely with each other and with law enforcement agencies. It facilitates early warning systems, such as broadcast fax, to alert local, state, and federal authorities and the media about urgent health threats and about the necessary prevention and response actions.

State Networks

In addition to the federal networks under the umbrella of the PHIN, there are state-level initiatives, for example:

- EpiCom in Florida (https://www.epicomfl.net/). Since early 2003, the Florida Department of Health has utilized an electronic information exchange and emergency alerting system, known as EpiCom, to provide an information exchange for the reporting and tracking of outbreaks and to alert public health officials of those events (Association of State and Territorial Health Officials [ASHTO], 2006).
- Kentucky Preparation and Response on Advanced Communications. Networks are also important for responding to public health emergencies. Response to Hurricane Katrina provided opportunities for new

public health communications systems to be tested. On September 7, 2005, the Kentucky Preparation and Response on Advanced Communications Technology (PROACT) network was activated to aid volunteer and evacuee coordination efforts. It connected 42 telehealth sites across the state in the first instance of PROACT's use during an actual public health emergency (ASHTO, 2006).

PUBLIC HEALTH INFORMATION SYSTEM: THE NEEDED SKILL SETS

This section addresses the information technology skill sets need to manage, access, and understand the wide variety of publically available surveillance and survey data. In addition, it provides insights in accessing electronic sources of knowledge. This section also addresses the challenges involved in developing and implementing information technology systems, with particular guidance on implementing syndrome surveillance systems and public health registry systems.

Using Databases: Medical Data Confidentiality and Privacy Legislation

Much of the data collected in surveys by NCHS and other organizations are personal data. The use of these data is carefully controlled to avoid invasions of privacy. Over the years, confidentiality protections have been enshrined in federal legislation—the Public Health Service Act of 1946, the Privacy Act of 1974, and the Health Insurance Portability and Accountability Act (HIPAA) of 1996. Public health professionals using or managing public health information technology systems should be acquainted with these federal laws and analogous statutes at the state level.

An *Assurance of Confidentiality* is a formal confidentiality protection authorized under Section 308(d) of the Public Health Service Act of 1946. It is used for projects conducted by the CDC that involve the collection or maintenance of sensitive identifiable or potentially identifiable information. This protection allows CDC programs to assure individuals and institutions involved in data collection projects that those conducting the project will protect the confidentiality of the data collected. The legislation states that no identifiable information may be used for any purpose other than the purpose for which it was supplied, unless such institution or individual has consented to that disclosure.

The Privacy Act of 1974, and its amendments, seek to regulate the collection, maintenance, use, and dissemination of personal information by federal executive branch agencies. The Privacy Act mandates that each federal agency have in place an administrative and physical security system to prevent the unauthorized release of personal records.

The Health Insurance Portability and Accountability Act (HIPAA) of 1996, among other things, set national standards for accessing and handling medical information. States are free to adopt laws that give *more* privacy, but state laws cannot take away the basic rights given by HIPAA. The act mandated the Department of Health and Human Services to draft a privacy regulation that was issued and became final on April 1, 2001. The regulation relates to "protected health information"; under HIPAA, this includes any individually identifiable health information, where *identifiable* includes not only data that are explicitly linked to a particular individual (e.g., Social Security number or telephone number), but also health information with data items that reasonably could be expected to allow individual identification. The regulation covers the use and disclosure of protected health information, accountability for this use and disclosure, and requirements for ensuring the security of protected health information.

Accessing the Data

Federal and state agencies that collect public health data usually publish reports that analyze the collected data. Public health professionals, however, often want to analyze the data in different ways than those included in the published reports. To facilitate this, many public agencies make the data available to the public. For example, over the years, the NCHS has released data for public use in several formats—IBM mainframe tapes, CD-ROMs, and downloadable files from the Internet. The NCHS is progressively moving to supporting one format— downloadable files from the Internet.

To preserve privacy and confidentiality, details that might identify or facilitate the identification of persons and organizations participating in NCHS surveys are suppressed in published data products. Despite the wide dissemination of NCHS data through publications and data releases, the inability to release files with sensitive variables limits the utility of NCHS data for research, policy, and programmatic purposes. In response to the public research community's interest in restricted data, the NCHS established the NCHS Research Data Center (RDC), a place where non-NCHS researchers can access detailed data files in a secure environment, without jeopardizing the confidentiality of respondents. The RDC provides restricted access to NCHS data either on site at NCHS locations or remotely (NCHS, 2008b).

Understanding Public Health Data Standards

Public health data standards facilitate public health data collection (e.g., at the point of care) in a consistent way across the nation and public health data reuse for multiple purposes (such as analysis of incidence rates and surveillance purposes). HIPAA greatly fostered the adoption and implementation of public health data standards by requiring the establishment of national standards for certain electronic healthcare insurance transactions. More recently, the Consolidated Health Informatics (CHI) initiative, one of 24 e-Gov (electronic government) initiatives established by President George W. Bush in 2001, led to the adoption of a portfolio of 20 electronic health messaging and terminology standards for use within the federal healthcare enterprise.

For public health professionals to use and exchange public health data, they must thoroughly understand the relevant data standards. The two key types of data standards are:

- *Terminologies*—the medical terms and concepts used to describe, classify, and code data elements and the data expression languages and syntax that describe the relationships among the terms/concepts (IOM, 2004). The following terminologies are important in public health:
  - ICD-CM: the International Classification of Diseases, Clinical Modification (discussed later).
  - SNOMED CT: Systemized Nomenclature of Medicine—Clinical Terms; a comprehensive clinical terminology developed to facilitate the electronic storage and retrieval of clinical information.
  - LOINC: Logical Observation Identifiers Names and Codes; facilitates the electronic transmission of laboratory results information to hospitals, ambulatory clinics, third-party payers, and other users of laboratory data.
  - NDC: National Drug Codes; the standard code set used to identify drugs and biologics marketed in the United States.
  - RxNorm; provides standard names for clinical drugs based on active ingredient, strength, and physical dose form.
- *Data interchange standards*—standard formats for electronically encoding the data elements (including sequencing and error handling). Interchange standards can also include document architectures for structuring data elements as they are exchanged and information models that define the relations among data elements (IOM, 2004). The following data interchange standards are important in public health:
  - HL7 Messaging Standard: Health level Seven; a standards organization that has developed a messaging standard for the electronic exchange of healthcare data.
  - ASC X12N Standards: Accredited Standards Committee (ASC) X12; develops standards for the elec-

tronic exchange of business data. The X12N sub-committee deals with electronic data interchange in the insurance industry, particularly as relating to health care.

The terminologies used for mortality, morbidity, and diagnosis are particularly import in public health:

- The International Statistical Classification of Diseases and Related Health Problems (usually abbreviated to International Classification of Diseases [ICD]) provides codes to classify diseases and a wide variety of signs, symptoms, external causes of injury or disease. The ICD, published by the World Health Organization, is used worldwide for morbidity and mortality statistics. The ICD is revised periodically and is currently in its 10th edition (ICD-10); ICD-11 is currently being planned. The United States began using ICD-10 to code and classify mortality data from death certificates in January 1999 for use by the National Center for Health Statistics.
- The International Classification of Diseases, Ninth Revision, Clinical Modification (ICD-9-CM) is based on the ICD-9. ICD-9-CM is used to assign codes to diagnoses associated with inpatient and outpatient visits in the United States and most National Center for Health Statistics (NCHS) surveys.
- ICD includes a set of mental disorders codes, but the American Psychiatric Association's (APA) Diagnostic and Statistical Manual of Mental Disorders (DSM) is the primary diagnostic system for psychiatric and psychological disorders within the United States. The current revision is DSM-IV published in 1994; DSM-V is currently being planned.

In using these and other code sets, it is important to know how the data were coded, why the data were coded, and the skill sets/training of the coders, because this may well affect the accuracy of the coding or may introduce bias into the coding—both important factors when using coded data for research purposes.

There are two important resources relating to public health data standards—the Public Health Data Standards Consortium (PHDSC) and the U.S. Health Information Knowledgebase (USHIK). The PHDSC is a standards organization focused on representing the public health community at the principal standards development organizations and promoting the use of data and systems standards by the public health community. The Consortium works with standards development organizations (e.g., HL7, X12) and data content committees (e.g., National Unified Content Committee [NUCC] and National Unified Billing Committee [NUBC])

to implement existing standards, to modify those standards to meet the needs of public health and research and, where appropriate, to develop new standards.

The USHIK is a health metadata registry funded and directed by the Agency for Healthcare Research and Quality in partnership with the Centers for Medicare & Medicaid Services (CMS). The USHIK provides and maintains a metadata registry of health information data element definitions, values, and information models that are available for browsing, comparison, synchronization, and harmonization purposes.

Analysis Tools

Once the reporting and survey data have been acquired by the public health researcher, there are a wide range of software packages available to carry out statistical analyses (for example, SAS/STAT and SPSS Statistics). Public health investigations have traditionally carried out geographic analyses of public health data. To aid this process, there are now available a wide range of GIS (Geographic Information System) software packages that utilize the ZIP code, address, or latitude/longitude of the public health event to display the location of events and to identify potentially important clusters.

Searching Electronic Knowledge Sources

There are three broad types of searching electronic knowledge sources—searching a database that uses a controlled vocabulary for indexing and searching (e.g., MEDLINE), searching a website created by a trustworthy organization, and Web searching using general search engines (e.g., Google).

MeSH and MEDLINE

The MeSH (Medical Subject Headings) vocabulary has been designed by the NLM for indexing and searching of the MEDLINE database using the PubMed retrieval tool (www.ncbi.nlm.nih.gov/sites/entrez?db=pubmed). The MeSH vocabulary consists of a tree structure with 16 main headings such as Anatomy (heading A), Diseases (heading C), Anthropology, Education, Sociology and Social Phenomena (heading I), and Health Care (heading N).

Each main heading is further defined, delineated, and broken down into more specific headings. For example, for Diseases (heading C), the next level begins:

Bacterial Infections and Mycoses (C01)
Virus Diseases (C02)
Parasitic Diseases (C03)

Each of these is broken down into more specific headings, and so on, for several more levels down.

The full set of headings (see www.nlm.nih.gov/mesh/trees2008.html.) is very extensive, and it is often quite difficult to know which MeSH terms to use. The NLM provides a MeSH Browser (www.nlm.nih.gov/mesh/MBrowser.html) to search for appropriate terms.

Another approach is to search for articles containing a key word or phrase in the journal title and/or abstract using the PubMed retrieval tool. Having found a few good journal articles, the researcher can look at the MeSH terms used in indexing these journal articles to identify the MeSH terms that can be used to retrieve further relevant articles.

Trustworthy Web Portals

General Web searching has its limitations (discussed later). There are, however, a wide range of trustworthy websites and Web portals (a website containing both articles and links to other websites). Examples include:

- The websites of state and federal agencies such as the Department of Health and Human Services (Healthfinder) and the National Institutes of Health (MedlinePlus).
- Portals such as Health Web (University of Michigan), HealthLinks (University of Washington), Health & Wellness (American Association of Retired Persons), and Health Insight (American Medical Association).
- Cochrane Collaboration (www.cochrane.org)—a database of systematic reviews of the literature on a wide range of medical topics.

It is good practice to identify a set of trustworthy websites and "bookmark" the addresses for easy access.

General Web Searching

General Web searching is convenient but full of pitfalls. The origin of the information provided is often unclear—is it an opinion, an interesting idea, or peer-reviewed research? Another factor to consider is the currency of the information; many websites are not routinely reviewed and updated. A further factor is the funder the Web site; commercial considerations might lead to the presentation of misleading or even inaccurate information.

There are organizations (e.g., Health on the Net Foundation, 2008) that provide a seal of approval for healthcare Web sites. This organization has developed a code of conduct (HONcode) to help standardize the reliability of Internet medical and health information. The code states that the site holds to a set of standards so that readers can know the source and purpose of the medical information presented. The standards cover the need to indicate the qualifications of the authors, to support information by references to source data, and for claims of benefits to be supported by balanced evi-

dence. No attempt is made to rate the veracity of the information provided.

Building and Managing Information Systems: Project Life Cycle

Most information technology projects, regardless of the type of application or industry, follow the same life cycle—a sequential set of phases that a system typically goes through—beginning with strategic business and information technology plans, followed by detailed requirements development, selecting the information technology system, implementation, post-implementation activities, and then, hopefully, after many years of useful life, the decision to replace the system.

Phase I: Strategic Business and Information Technology Plans

The first phase is the development of the strategic objectives of the (public health) organization, which lies outside the scope of this chapter. Arising directly from the strategic business plan, the strategic information technology plan is an inventory of information technology initiatives needed to achieve the strategic business objectives. These initiatives could include new systems, modifications to existing systems, or major enhancements to the organization's infrastructure of software, computers, and networks. The information technology strategy should contain a timeline of the required investments, a high-level statement of the budget requirements, and an overview of the major risks and risk-management options.

Phase II: Detailed Requirements Development

Once a business case has been made for a particular application (e.g., the implementation of a registry), the detailed requirements must be determined. A project steering group will be needed, ideally consisting of five to seven people, although often such steering groups are much larger to accommodate all the interested parties. The steering group should include all the key stakeholders—users, information technology staff, and senior management. This group might also include an external expert with experience in designing and implementing a similar application in other organizations. After identifying the needs of users and researching similar applications in other organizations (e.g., by making site visits), the group should craft a set of requirements covering:

- The data needed and how they will be acquired.
- How the quality of the data to be used will be reviewed and the rules for rejecting or changing data.
- Links to other computer systems for sending and receiving data.

- The functional tasks required by each type of user.
- The data and access security needs and system availability requirements.
- The help functions to be embedded within the application.
- The hardware and software environment in which the system will be implemented.

The end result of this process will be a detailed document covering these topics.

Phase III: Selecting the Information Technology System

The next step in the selection of the information technology solution is to draw up a list of products/companies that could satisfy the requirements. This usually involves a review of the trade literature, holding discussions with possible vendors, and visits to successful implementations. Other issues that need to be considered are the maturity of the software product and the long-term viability of the software vendor. Once a short-list of products/companies has been established, the detailed statement of requirements should be sent out to those on the list.

The system selection team should be made up of users and information technology staff and have credibility within the organization. Each vendor's response to the statement of requirements should be carefully reviewed to determine the vendor's compliance with each detailed point on the requirement. Following up with each vendor's reference sites (or with other sites not provided by the vendor) is important to get a sense of how satisfied current users are with the vendor's product and its implementation of that product.

Once a vendor is chosen, the next step is contract negotiation. This covers a wide range of activities beyond the initial cost and ongoing maintenance charges, including the implementation timetable, the schedule for testing the product once implemented, the training and help desk services to be provided by the vendor, penalties for late implementation, and the staff that the vendor will commit to the implementation.

Phase IV: Implementation

In many ways, this is the most crucial phase, because this is the first time the whole user community becomes involved, most of whom have had little or no involvement so far with the project. As with other phases of the project, this phase must be carefully planned, with the plan communicated to the user community. The implementation begins with the testing of the product software, followed by user training for the new system. Prior to the system going live, user expectations will have to be managed because users will almost certainly have to alter the way they work. The necessary training should be made available. User resistance to the required changes in their work processes could doom the whole implementation. Throughout the implementation phase, it is important to keep communicating with the users on progress and to respond rapidly to user problems as they occur.

Phase V: Post-Implementation Activities

Immediately following implementation, it is important to make sure the system is being used in the planned way. More user training may be necessary at this stage. Any system problems must be rapidly identified and addressed.

After a period of successful operation, the contract with the vendor should be reviewed and final payments made. Arrangements should then made to establish a process for making changes to the system to meet changing business needs and for incorporating software upgrades provided by the vendor. In addition, the organization should participate in external user groups (activities sometimes provided by the software vendor) to learn how others are using the product and how they have overcome any problems.

Phase VI: Starting Again

The final phase is the decision to replace the system with another system. This may be necessary because the current system no longer has the needed functionality, the current software is expensive to maintain or is no longer being supported by the software vendor, or much better software systems are now available. The whole cycle now begins again with the strategic business and information technology plans phase.

Information Technology Projects Are Challenging

The implementation of an information technology system is challenging, and a large proportion of information technology projects are failures. Charrette (2005) identified a number of factors, either individually or jointly, that can lead to failure:

- *Lack of senior management commitment*—failing to commit sufficient money and appropriate personnel, or not realizing the impact of the project's impact on the organization's business.
- *Bad management decisions* (the single greatest cause of project failure)—engaging the wrong type of staff, choosing the wrong type of software package, or failing to identify and respond to the risks associated with the project.
- *Being seduced by overhyped new technologies*—innovative or immature technologies are particularly hard to implement.

- *Too much complexity*—complex projects are impossible to thoroughly test.
- *Sloppy project development and implementation practices.*
- *Failure to confront reality*—having an organizational culture that is not ready to implement the information technology project.

Successful implementation involves careful planning, an enthusiastic implementation team, and avoidance of the preceding pitfalls.

Implementing Syndrome Surveillance Systems

The key function of a syndrome surveillance system is the detection of potential health threats—unusually high numbers of occurrences of events of interest to the public health community. There are an emerging number of detection systems: RODS (Real-time Outbreak Detection System), developed by the University of Pittsburgh; EARS (Early Aberration Reporting System), developed by the CDC; and the Electronic Surveillance System for Early Notification of Community-based Epidemics, developed by Johns Hopkins University.

Mandl et al. (2004) provide guidance on implementing a syndrome surveillance system. Assuming that the diseases to be detected and the corresponding syndromes to be tracked have been decided upon, here are a number of key steps:

- Identify the data sources to be used. Outbreaks of a disease may lead to purchases of over-the-counter medications, school/work absenteeism, and encounters with the healthcare system (e.g., primary care or emergency department visits). The most valuable data sources are those that are electronically stored, allow robust syndrome groupings, and are available in a timely fashion.
- Group the data in a way that provides information useful to public health professionals. Experience has shown that healthcare encounter data such as ICD-9 diagnosis code and chief complaint can be mapped onto syndromes. It is important to be aware that substantial variations in ICD-9 coding quality across healthcare institutions are possible.
- Healthcare organizations that generate the data for use in syndrome surveillance systems are likely to use a wide variety of computer systems. For data coding and data exchange, public healthcare data standards should be adopted (see the earlier section on public healthcare data standards).
- To demonstrate the validity of a potential health threat often requires more detailed examination of the clinical data of the patients involved—thus, appropriate extra data should be ingested as part of the original encounter data.

- Finally, the confidentiality of surveillance data from individuals must be protected. HIPAA regulations and the relevant state statutes must be adhered to.

Implementing Registries

The California HealthCare Foundation has recently published two monographs on disease registries—one covers the use of disease registries (Metzger, 2004) and the other evaluates 16 free and commercially available registry software applications (Simon and Powers, 2004). Both provide valuable insights into implementing all types of registries, not just disease registries. Key issues that need to be addressed during the implementation of a registry are as follows:

- Precisely define the business rules for including a patient in the registry and for amending/updating data on an existing patient.
- Carefully consider what data should be collected for each patient. The challenge is not to collect too much data initially—start with a basic set and add secondary data later.
- Capture data electronically whenever possible—clinicians do not want to enter data manually into registries.
- Institute procedures (automatic if possible) for judging whether a patient has been correctly included in the registry and for checking the quality of data collected for each patient (e.g., is the patient's weight consistent with the patient's age?).
- Design the key set of analyses that need to be carried out—again, start small, adding further types of analyses later.
- Identify the roles with regard to the registry (i.e., read-only access, read/write access) for each type of user—clinician, public health researcher, registry administrator.

CONCLUSION

In the coming years, public health managers and leaders will need to address a broader range of challenges without a commensurate increase in the public health workforce. Innovative strategies will be needed to counter these shortages of resources. Public health informatics has an important role to play in developing such innovative strategies. Building information technology systems is challenging. Achieving the full benefits of investments in information technology requires public health managers and leaders to be information technology literate with an understanding of how to use and implement public health information technology systems.

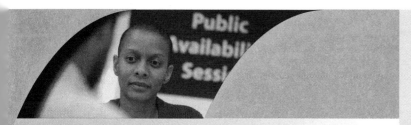

Discussion Questions

1. In what ways can information technology support public health activities?

2. How can registries help improve public health?

3. What are the key issues in searching for trustworthy public health information?

4. Why are public health data standards important?

5. Why are telecommunications networks becoming increasingly important in public health?

6. What are the main challenges involved in implementing public health information technology projects?

REFERENCES

ASTHO (Association of State and Territorial Health Officials). *Issue Brief: Health Information Technology in Public Health Emergencies.* Washington, DC: ASTHO; 2006.

Bradley CA, et al. BioSense: Implementation of a National Early Event Detection and Situational Awareness System. *Morb Mortal Wkly Rep.* August 2005;54(Suppl):11–19.

Charrette RN. Why Software Fails. *Spectrum Online.* September 2005.

CDC Solutions. *BioSense: Real-Time Biosurveillance.* 2008. http://www.cdc.gov/phin/library/documents/pdf/111759_biosense2.pdf. Accessed July 25, 2008.

Federal Register. *Agency Forms Undergoing Paperwork Reduction Act Review. Vol. 72(220). Notices, 64229-64230:* Department of Health and Human Services, Centers for Disease Control and Prevention; November 15, 2007.

Freedman MA, Weed JA. The National Vital Statistics System. In: O'Carroll PW, Yasnoff WA, Ward MA, Ripp LH, Martin EL, eds. *Public Health Informatics and Information Systems.* New York: Springer; 2003.

Health on the Net Foundation. 2008. HON Code of Conduct (HONcode) for medical and health Web sites. Available: http://www.hon.ch/HONcode/Conduct.html. Accessed July 25, 2008.

Heffernan R, et al. Syndromic Surveillance in Public Health Practice, New York City. *Emerging Infectious Diseases.* 2004;10(5):858–864.

Heitz R. Wisconsin's Immunization Registry. *Wisconsin Medical Journal.* 2005;104(5):83–85.

Hersh WR. *Information Retrieval: A Health Care Perspective.* New York: Springer-Verlag; 1996.

IOM (Institute of Medicine). *To Err Is Human: Building a Safer Health Care System.* Washington, DC: National Academy Press; 2000.

IOM (Institute of Medicine). *Patient Safety: Achieving a New Standard for Care.* Washington, DC: The National Academies Press; 2004.

IOM (Institute of Medicine). *PEPFAR Implementation: Progress and Promise.* Washington, DC: The National Academies Press; 2007.

Loonsk JW, et al. The Public Health Information Network (PHIN) Preparedness Initiative. *J Am Med Inform Assoc.* 2006;13(1):1–5.

Mandl KD, et al. Implementing Syndromic Surveillance: A Practical Guide Informed by Early Experience. *J Am Med Inform Assoc.* 2004;11(2):141–150.

McHugh LA, et al. Effect of Electronic Laboratory Reporting on the Burden of Lyme Disease Surveillance—New Jersey, 2001–2006. *Morb Mortal Wkly Rep.* January 2008;57(2):42–45.

Metzger, J. 2004. *Using Computerized Registries in Chronic Disease Care.* Oakland, CA: California HealthCare Foundation.

MMWR (Morbidity and Mortality Weekly Report). 2005. Progress in Improving State and Local Disease Surveillance—United States, 2000–2005. 54(33):822–825.

NASHP (National Academy for State Health Policy). 2008. Patient Safety Toolbox for States. Available: http://www.psa.state.pa.us/psa/cwp/view.asp?a=1293&q=445966&psaNav=l. Accessed July 25, 2008.

NCHS (National Center for Health Statistics). 2008a. Available: http://www.cdc.gov/nchs/about.htm. Accessed July 25, 2008.

NCHS. 2008b. National Center for Health Statistics, Research Data Center: Guidelines for Proposal Submission (Last revised: June 6, 2008). Available: http://www.cdc.gov/nchs/data/r&d/Guidelines060408.pdf. Accessed August 7, 2008.

O'Carroll PW. Introduction to Public Health Informatics. In: O'Carroll PW, Yasnoff WA, Ward MA, Ripp LH, Martin EL, eds. *Public Health Informatics and Information Systems.* New York: Springer; 2003.

PA-DOH (Pennsylvania Department of Health). 2008. Pennsylvania's National Electronic Disease Surveillance System (PA-NEDSS). Available: http://www.dsf.health.state.pa.us/health/cwp/view.asp?Q=230681. Accessed August 4, 2008.

PA-PSRS (Pennsylvania Patient Safety Reporting System). 2008. Patient Safety Advisories. Available: http://www.psa.state.pa.us/psa/cwp/view.asp?a=1293&q=445966&psaNav=l. Accessed July 25, 2008.

Roush S, et al. Mandatory Reporting of Diseases and Conditions by Health Care Professionals and Laboratories. *JAMA.* 1999;282:164–170.

Simon J, Powers M. *Chronic Disease Registries: A Product Review.* Oakland, CA: California HealthCare Foundation; 2004.

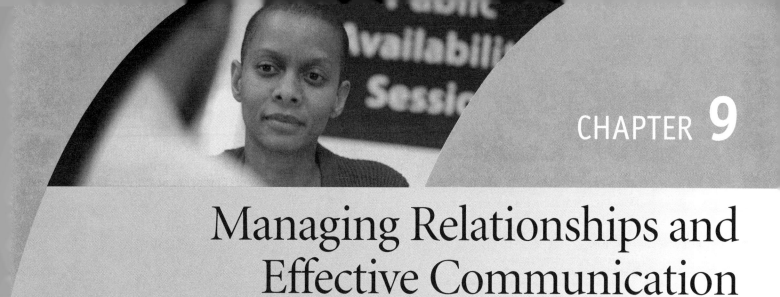

CHAPTER **9**

Managing Relationships and Effective Communication

Blaine Parrish and Robert E. Burke

INTRODUCTION

Managing relationships as a public health leader, manager, and practitioner is no different than managing relationships as any other business professional. Creating, maintaining, and rebuilding relationships among the diverse public health professionals, however, requires a set of interrelated, complicated, and multifaceted endeavors. Many public health practitioners have been labeled as "difficult" because they seek perfection through their exceptional training, and they compete fiercely in a domain that demands a highly intelligent cohort (Preston, 2005). Public health professionals rely heavily on myriad people with different educational levels, who work in different roles and positions. The professionals include members of the board of directors, skilled senior managers, hard-working front-line employees, specialists trained in a particular health issue or business management skill, consultants who offer expertise when needed, volunteers, consumers of the programs or products being used, and leaders of the communities in which these individuals work, receive services, and/or live. Each relationship plays an important part in developing public health infrastructure, establishing health programs, implementing health policy, and disseminating educational programs for a strong public health system. In this chapter, we examine what is necessary for these leaders and managers to work with these seemingly discordant individuals and to communicate effectively within the public health arena.

Effective communication is the key to keeping these relationships positive and ensuring that information needed within the organization or community flows quickly and efficiently up and down the communication line. Each relationship demands its own type of communication and monitoring. We explain how to manage these relationships for two reasons: (1) so that public health and better healthcare messages are clear to the community, and (2) so that consistent messages are reinforced both through and within the organization.

Several themes emerge when managers balance the needs of the community with the needs of individuals:

- Managing relationships and communicating effectively are more natural and/or easier for some individuals than others.
- Training managers and leaders to be effective in building relationships and to develop strong communication skills is essential, but it cannot take the place of practical experience.
- Understanding the basic types of organization within the public healthcare system and who works in these organizations is essential.
- Building relationships through open communication allows managers and leaders to stay involved with the most important aspects of public health infrastructure, including: planning/organizing, staffing/directing, managing change, decision making/problem solving, and motivating/communicating (Koontz & O'Donnell, 1972).

Vital to building lasting positive relationships and advancing management of public health is the ability of a community to recruit natural leaders, managers with practical experience, and individuals with specific business/public health training, then to use their collective knowledge and experience to maintain the system.

LEARNING OBJECTIVES

After reading this chapter, the reader will be able to:

1 Define what types of leaders and managers are in public health and how the type of leader one is affects how relationships are maintained.

2. Understand which relationships leaders and managers need to manage in order to function in a public health system.

3. Apply principles of management to developing relationships and effective communication.

4. Communicate leadership and management issues using appropriate channels and technologies/techniques.

MANAGEMENT FRAMEWORK

As presented in Chapter 2, Henri Fayol was an important figure in the development of modern concepts of management functions. Fayol's division of these functions into five areas—planning, organizing, commanding, coordinating, and controlling—is evident in organizational charts, strategic planning documents, quality improvement and assurance plans, grant applications, and other written materials in public health (Fayol, 1949). Each function is a vital building block in the development of a public health system and the management of that system. But, since Fayol's early research, the U.S. work-force has changed—making understanding why they do what they do as important as doing what they do.

In addition to Fayol, Frederick Taylor contributed to an equally important concept of scientific management, a concept that includes analysis of workflow to improve productivity. This concept is still very much alive in public health, most prominently with hospitals and nursing (Grabin, 2007). But while we can learn much about the productivity of individual workers and dividing up responsibilities, these models do not help leaders and managers communicate or manage relationships. Critics argue that division of labor actually dehumanizes workers and promotes an "us versus them" mentality (Catton, 1985). When individuals worked on the assembly line, only productivity (how fast the product could be made, the minimum amount of resources necessary to produce the product, what minimum standards could be set for workers to keep disruption of production to a minimum) mattered to management. Now, employee protections, a more educated workforce, and the nature of current business practices make management and communication skills more important in motivating the workforce.

Study **Figure 9-1**. Notice how the functions of a public health department are organized into areas of common interest, expertise, and public health priorities and then controlled

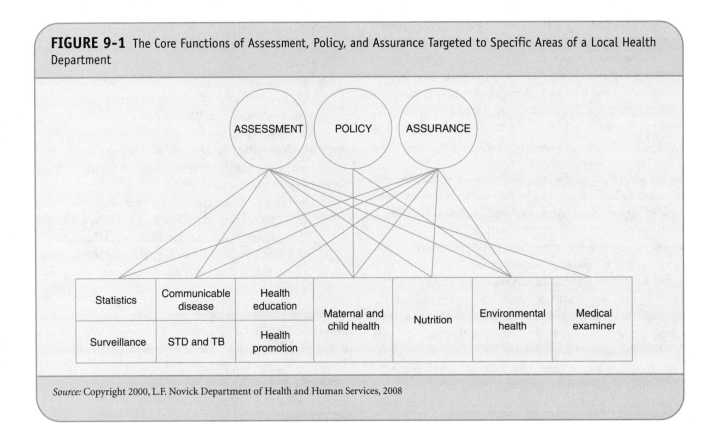

FIGURE 9-1 The Core Functions of Assessment, Policy, and Assurance Targeted to Specific Areas of a Local Health Department

Source: Copyright 2000, L.F. Novick Department of Health and Human Services, 2008

and coordinated across these areas through filters such as assessment, policy, and assurance. These functions are important because a leader or manager must have the ability to look within these groups and tailor communication and relationship building based on the interests of the individuals and key stakeholders within these groups. This is no assembly line.

Individuals within each function or area has expertise and information to share with peers, individuals from other areas, and managers—all working together to maintain a system that relies on a strong coordinating effort.

Now study **Figure 9-2** and compare it with Figure 9-1. Notice how the lines in the organizational chart are more

FIGURE 9-2

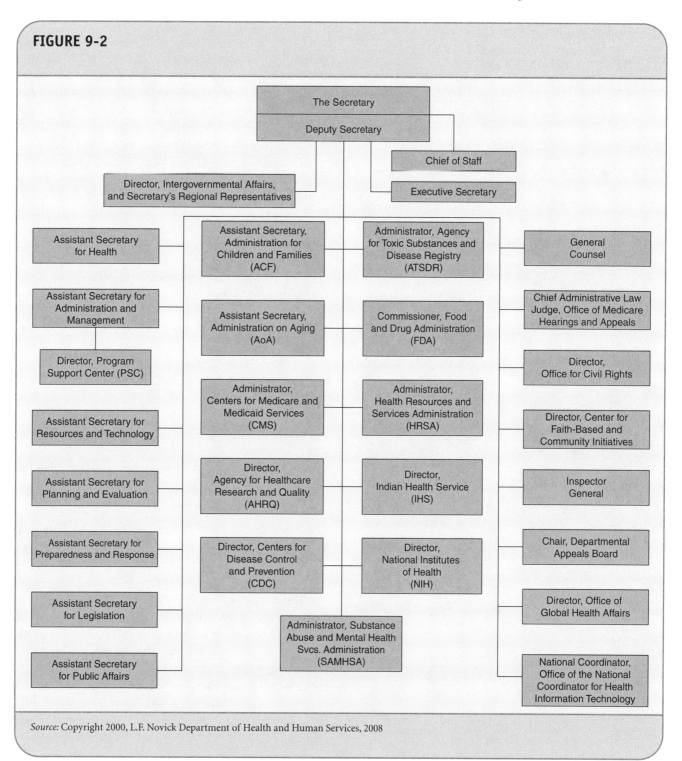

Source: Copyright 2000, L.F. Novick Department of Health and Human Services, 2008

specific and hierarchical. Within this system, individuals are listed by their title, not by their function. They are represented in relationship to those "above and below" them with a strict interpretation of the relationship between and among the individuals. Leaders and managers must also manage these more individual and personal relationships—a different skill than managing communication and relationships with an entire group as illustrated in Figure 9-1.

RELATIONSHIP MANAGEMENT

Before discussing the types of relationships that a leader/manager must manage, it is important to understand what types of leaders and managers are in public health and how the type of leader affects how relationships are maintained.

Primal Leadership

Natural leadership can also be defined as *primal leadership*. A two-year study by researchers Goleman, Boyatzis, and McKee (2004) led them to contend that the success of communication and motivation in an organization depends on the mood and behaviors of the leader. "A cranky and ruthless boss creates a toxic organization of negative underachievers; an upbeat and inspirational leader spawns acolytes for whom any challenge is surmountable" (*Harvard Business Review*, 1979). We all have individuals in our lives who do not have to work hard to motivate us or to deflate us. These individuals have a natural way with communication—a way to almost instantly assess our mood or our position and to either help us resolve issues or make us feel like we are not capable of functioning successfully.

Public health practitioners are under extreme daily pressures. Providing direct healthcare services, juggling limited resources, and making decisions on which programs continue or which programs are cut, among other issues, make the perfectionism found in public health leaders and managers manifest itself in different ways. Natural leaders with a positive outlook can move with the tide and manage relationships because they have built trust based on the consistency of their positive mood and behaviors. Those with a negative outlook only increase frustration and mistrust and cause workers—and the community at large—to doubt the motives of the leader or the manager's commitment to the public health issue (Goleman et al., 2004).

Taught Leadership

Can leadership be taught? Consider what David Halberstam (2004) says about leaders:

> The truth is that in most fields, it's a natural process. Leaders are men and women who have

chosen the right profession. They're good at it, and because they're good at it, they like it, and because they like it, they're even better at it. They're so good at it that they'd rather work than play. They're naturals, and excelling comes naturally as well. They've understood their field from the start, and they've studied it without even knowing they've studied it.

So if we like what we do, are good at it, and would rather work than play, are we a leader? Dr. Keith Grint (2000) from the University of Oxford suggests the "most useful way for organizations to view leadership is as an art not a science, as a collective process not an individual achievement, and that the most successful leaders lead through negotiations not logic."

Developed by the Robert Wood Johnson Foundation, Turning Point's mission is to strengthen collaboration among community-based public health programs. Under the initiative, Dr. Carl Larson, University of Denver, developed six modules to train individuals to bring this concept to the community:

- *Assessing the environment for collaboration:* understanding the context for change before you act.
- *Creating clarity—visioning and mobilizing:* defining shared values and engaging people in positive action.
- *Building trust:* creating safe places for developing shared purpose and action.
- *Sharing power and influence:* developing the synergy of people, organizations, and communities to accomplish more.
- *Developing people:* committing to the development of people as your key asset through mentoring and coaching.
- *Self-reflection—personal continuous quality improvement (CQI):* understanding your own leadership, engaging others (Turning Point, 2006).

Notice how different these six concepts are from Taylorism. The leader/manager is actually responsible for maintaining a relationship with the workers and must rely on them as a key component to success.

This managing of relationships is important, especially in light of a 1988 Institute of Medicine (IOM) report suggesting that more focus needs to be on developing leaders in public health. Some skeptics maintain that leaders are born, not raised. The type of leadership training suggested by the report, however, is one that takes the best of the individual leader or manager and, as Larson suggests, "shift[s] from authority-focused leadership to collaborative and team-oriented leadership" and combines that "with adequate leadership education and training" (Larson et al., 2002). Leaders with the capacities and characteristics consistent with this more collaborative approach are essential and can play an important part in the development of a successful public health organization, program, or system.

THE COLLECTIVE PROCESS OF LEADERSHIP

The idea that leadership is a collective process is one that we explore throughout this chapter. Because leadership is something that has been defined as both natural and taught, let us focus on the collective process of leadership—and explore the relationships that must be managed for success.

The Challenges of Managing Different Groups

Being managed is not something most individuals have on their to-do list. Leaders and managers know that there are challenges managing any group. What about the twenty-somethings? "They're ambitious, they're demanding and they question everything, so if there isn't a good reason for that long commute or late night, don't expect them to do it. When it comes to loyalty, the companies they work for are last on their list—behind their families, their friends, their communities, their co-workers and, of course, themselves" (Hira, 2007). True or not, these perceptions are exactly the information that leaders and managers must have to successfully engage in a collective process of leadership.

Public health leaders and managers must work with individuals from many different types of organizations: for-profit; not-for-profit; local, state, or federal agencies; and private–public partnerships. For-profit public health organizations may answer to shareholders and a board of directors, which must always look to the bottom line to measure success. Not-for-profit organizations may spend as much time searching for funding as they do providing public health services within the community. Local, state, and federally funded and/or administered public health programs exist within the confines of ever-changing public health priorities based on the currently elected leadership. Private–public partnerships strive to join the best in private best practices (management, service delivery, etc.) with the resources and vast delivery system of the public sector.

While the organizations may differ in their business structure, they are all staffed with the same basic personnel: a board of directors, senior managers, front-line employees, specialists trained in particular health issues or business skills, consultants, and volunteers. Although consumers and community leaders are not staff members, managing these relationships are equally important to success.

Understanding and Communication

The Leadership Practices Inventory (LPI) provides a framework for understanding and communicating with all the stakeholders in an organization or system. The LPI is a 360-degree management assessment tool to help leaders define their behaviors and use various workshops and programs to gain a set of behaviors that will facilitate better understanding and communication. These behaviors include:

- *Model the way*: finding a way to clarify personal values and set examples by aligning actions and shared values.
- *Inspire a shared vision*: imagining possibilities for the future and enlisting others in the common vision by appealing to shared goals and objectives.
- *Challenge the process*: seeking innovative ways to change, grow, and improve through risk-taking and experimentation—learning from mistakes and celebrating small victories.
- *Enable others to act*: fostering collaboration and promoting goals and trust among individuals and organization—uplifting others through shared power.
- *Encourage the heart*: recognizing contributions and showing appreciation for excellence by celebrating values and victories to create a sprit of community (Kouzes & Posner, 1997).

Each of these behaviors becomes the cornerstone for interacting with the individuals and/or organizations that make up the system. Notice how different behaviors are necessary to manage the relationships with the various types of individuals.

Governing Boards

The governing board of an organization is responsible for the oversight of the mission of the organization and to offer advice in meeting the goals and objectives of the organization. A leader's responsibility, in many cases a chief executive officer (CEO) or chief financial officer (CFO), is to manage this relationship by defining a line of responsibility so the governing board does not become a micromanaging group. Managing this relationship takes recognizing the political nature of some governing bodies.

Individuals are chosen for the governing board because of their expertise in the area; because of friendships or relationships with major funders or donors; by nomination of the CEO or executive director and, therefore, because of a possible relationship with that person; and finally because one is a member of the organization's staff or a consumer of the products/services provided by the organization. Each person on the governing board may have aligned or competing ideas of how the organization should be led and managed. Managing these relationships means inspiring a shared vision. It also requires modeling "the way" so the governing board understands how the leader envisions their interaction and responsibilities in light of the day-to-day responsibilities the organization's staff has for completing the mission.

Because the governing board has responsibility for evaluating the performance of the leader, the relationship between the manager and the board must be expertly maintained by an individual who can both hold a firm line and build trust and consensus. This can only be accomplished through experience, open communication, and staying true to the mission of the organization (Charan, 2006).

Senior Managers

Like a governing board, a senior management team is comprised of a number of very different individuals. A leader can get to know all the individuals but can never meet the expectations of everyone. These senior managers will have their own goals—advancement, retirement, maintaining the status quo, "mixing things up," etc. The challenge for the leader is to share the path for success through development and implementation of a roadmap. The key to managing relationships with senior management is to keep them involved and active in the process. Ongoing support of the team is vital to getting the message out to the larger organization and getting the work done. The leader must be honest and up-front about the challenges and benefits of completing certain tasks and must provide the necessary resources so the senior managers know they are supported and respected.

All five LPI behaviors are essential in this setting to manage relationships with senior management. Again, inspiring a shared vision (getting buy-in from senior leadership) and modeling the way (patterning communication style and personal interest in workers' output) are the vital components of managing this relationship.

Front-line Employees

Front-line workers receive a significant amount of discussion in management and leadership literature. Why shouldn't they? Without them, the hour-by-hour work of an organization would not get accomplished, and the mission of the organization would not be realized. Nurses, social or case workers, van drivers, cashiers, administrative assistants, and others face the public on a daily basis and feel the immediate reaction of implemented programs, cutbacks, policies, and other organizational or programmatic decisions. One major factor is front and center when managing these relationships—time. Managers need to see what the front-line staff does and ap-

preciate what it takes to be out in the public eye minute-by-minute. These individuals need to know that leaders and managers are with them, understand the job they do, and are sympathetic to the challenges they face.

Enabling others to act and modeling the way are two behaviors that can help front-line workers better relate to the leader and/or manager. When employees feel they have the resources they need and the process is concrete, they respond by being satisfied that someone cares about their experience. In addition, when the "boss" is willing to get his or her hands dirty by helping out when work needs to be done, these workers develop a respect for the leader, rather than imagining him or her sitting in a big office, kicked back in a leather chair enjoying a cigar while everyone else is "working."

Trained Specialists

Defining "trained specialist" is not difficult. Think of the 25- to 35-year-old information technology (IT) person sitting down the hall who types undecipherable lines of characters into a computer, which in turn become Web pages. Think of the person on the second floor who day-in and day-out operates a machine that takes "slice" pictures of a patient's brain. These individuals are trained to do something that you may understand in the abstract but could not perform as a regular part of your responsibilities. How does one manage a relationship with someone who does something that is a mystery?

Managing this relationship means acknowledging the special nature of the work the specialist does and taking an interest in the work by learning the special skills or terms (lingo) that will help ease communication. Specialists may not have breadth of knowledge, and the leader/manager can assist the specialist by providing mentors to give them a better understanding of the entire organization. They, in turn, can help the leader/manager better understand their function by using the depth of their knowledge in one area to share a vision of new things that are possible for the organization.

Consultants

Consultants should do just that—consult; that is, they should bring new or at least different ideas to the organization, not manage their implementation. Today, the consultant is more of an independent contractor. What is the difference to a leader or manager? It depends on the nature of the work the consultant is doing. There are several reasons to hire a consultant: the need for additional skills current employees do not have; the need for intelligent advice, which will assist the leader/manager in making a decision; getting an outside perspective so there is a fresh look at the issue; and the need for limited commitment, which allows the organization to let the consultant go after his or her services are no longer needed. If expectations are not managed—for example, when the consultant expects just to give advice and the organization expects the consultant to do the work—the relationship can quickly turn sour.

Managing these relationships can be easy or quite difficult—and mostly depends on the work of the consultant. The benefit is that the consultant has limited time with the organization, so communication can be honest, direct, and immediate. If the consultant is good, the communication will also be good. The relationship becomes difficult is when the consultant is not up to the task, does not have the skills advertised, and/or was selected primarily because of a personal relationship with someone at the organization. These confounding factors can muddle communication, cause work product to suffer, and cause permanent staff to resent the money being paid to the consultant when work is not being produced or is being produced poorly. Leaders and managers must be direct in what is expected and hold the consultant to the highest standards. Future work and a beneficial relationship to both parties depend on the management of expectations. The expectations should be discussed and agreed upon before entering into a contract.

Volunteers

For some organizations, volunteers are one of the reason employees are not overworked and that services get delivered on time or in an efficient way. In a time of budget cuts, reduced donations, and staff shortages, the volunteers fill in—free of charge—to make sure the consumers' needs are met and the organization can continue to function. Managing this relationship takes an incredible amount of encouraging the heart. Leaders and managers must show volunteers that they are appreciated, they must be given uncharacteristic flexibility in work responsibilities, and yet they must be held to a standard that does not compromise staff morale or quality of services. The bane of any organization is the unhappy volunteer. What can a leader do? A favorite phrase for volunteers is, "You can't fire a volunteer!" In fact, many volunteers are "fired" by reducing their hours worked or shifting their responsibilities. Volunteers are no different than paid staff in that they must have a strong work ethic and the ability to get the work done in order to fit into the organization.

The vast majority of volunteers are hard working, responsible, and responsive to the leadership and workers at the organization. The leader/manager can use all behaviors of leadership used with front-line staff. Volunteers need to know that they are useful, that they can provide input that will be taken seriously, that they have a stake in what is being provided to consumers, and most importantly, that their free time

is not taken for granted (i.e., the leader/manager is sitting around and getting paid while the volunteers are working like crazy for free). Managing these relationships also takes common sense—if it were you volunteering, what would you expect? Like being in the place of the consumer, leaders and managers can benefit from putting themselves in the place of the volunteer—making it easier to communicate with them.

Consumers

In public health, consumers are usually individuals who are served by one or more of the primary healthcare or ancillary services provided by the organization. When consumers are happy with their services, the leader or manager may never hear anything—including positive feedback about the program or the staff. Organizations that conduct needs assessments or satisfaction surveys usually find that when services are being provided in a competent, accessible way, consumers are happy and content. However, when consumers are unhappy, everyone from front-line staff to the governing board usually hears about the issues. Consumers write letters, make phone calls, attend board meetings, and talk within the community about their displeasure.

It is a mistake to leave dealing with unhappy consumers to front-line staff or senior managers. This is an opportunity for the leader to involve the consumer in making the process better. The leader can challenge the process, look at it from the consumers' perspectives, and use the information to feed back into the behaviors of inspiring a shared vision and enabling others to act. Managing this relationship takes courage and personal involvement—nothing short of getting out of the business environment and seeing the organization through different eyes. While a leader and/or manager cannot completely disassociate him- or herself from being the leader, he or she can work to understand how the consumer must feel, based on walking through the program or service with that person. To the consumer, that simple act shows an amount of compassion and interest that may go a long way to easing unhappiness and inspiring the consumer to become more involved in his or her own care.

Community Leaders/Other Organizations

An organization's reputation is always at stake in a community, based on what the organization and the leadership do in the community. Sometimes organizations collaborate to meet the needs of the community. Sometimes organizations must compete for funding, volunteers, and even consumers to be successful and to meet their individuals needs and continue to maintain and build their own infrastructure. How a leader/manager manages these relationships reflects on the organization and all those associated with it. While leaders and managers of other organizations may be willing to work with you, there is no way to know everything that motivates them—their system is equal to yours with its own challenges and pressures. The best way to manage these relationships is to inspire other leaders to meet their own goals and the goals of their organization, while enabling them to meet their goals—and you to meet yours—by acting in a collective best interest to serve the community. The best of public health happens in collaboration with those we compete against and those we depend on. In most communities, these are one and the same.

Community leaders—those who may be elected or self-appointed to watch over the well-being of the community—are sometimes a challenge to relate to. Your domain may be bigger or smaller than their influence, but community leaders have a way of deciding for themselves what interests they should take on and which ones they will leave alone. Whatever their motivation, listening to their interests, their ideas, and their demands will only benefit you. A good leader listens first and reacts second (Rynders, 1999).

CONCLUSION

This chapter has presented several distinct methods and ideas to demonstrate that managing relationships as a public health leader, manager, and practitioner is no different than managing relationships as any other business professional. Public health professionals work with and rely heavily on myriad people with different educational levels and who work in different roles and positions. Effective communication is the key to keeping these relationships positive and ensuring that information needed within the organization or community flows quickly and efficiently up and down the communication line. Each relationship demands its own type of communication and monitoring.

Managing relationships is ultimately a shared responsibility—a collaboration. Leaders and managers cannot manage these relationships without active participation from senior managers, front-line staff, specialists, consultants, volunteers, consumers, and community leaders. Management and leadership training must not take the place of meetings between leaders/managers and those they work with. In order for leaders and managers to be successful, they must rely on these relationships—as much as those working for the leader and manager must rely on these relationships to collectively meet the mission of the organization.

Effective communication is the tool to make these relationships work. Every LPI behavior discussed is a communication avenue to make sharing information, understanding motivations, accomplishing tasks, and ultimately serving the public a reality.

Case Example

On July 3, 2002, Julie Gerberding, MD, MPH, was appointed head of the Centers for Disease Control and Prevention. Dr. Gerberding had previously served as Acting Deputy Director of the National Centers for Infectious Diseases (NCID) and led the CDC's response to the anthrax bioterrorism scare in 2001. After becoming director of the CDC, Dr. Gerberding began implementing the "Futures Initiative," which would have moved the current 12 subdivisions into four coordinating centers. The idea turned out to be wildly unpopular. With 37% of the CDC's 8,500 employees responding to an anonymous online survey, two-thirds of those responding opposed the reorganization plan. Employees sited as their main objections: "an 'inappropriate' business focus to the public health mission of CDC, low employee morale, increased bureaucracy, loss of trust, loss of important staff members, and damage to the reputation of the agency" (Kaiser Daily Health Policy Report, 2005).

Following the announcement of the reorganization, four former directors of the National Institute of Occupational Safety and Health (NIOSH) wrote a letter voicing concern about the reorganization plan (Kaiser Daily Health Policy Report, 2004). Dr. James Hughes, the Center for Infectious Diseases director, and Dr. Harold Marolis, the chief of the viral hepatitis division for 17 years, both resigned because of the focus on reorganization rather than on scientific inquiry. Their resignations meant that six of the eight department heads at the time had resigned. Dr. Gerberding is the first female director of the CDC; all four former directors of NIOSH and all those who have resigned are male. A controversial statement made in 2005 by Harvard University's President Howard Summers ignited a national conversation about the role of women in science and math. Summers stated that "innate differences between men and women might be one reason fewer women succeed in science and math careers" (Bombardieri, 2005). Dr. Gerberding herself, in response to the statement, recounted her own discrimination:

There was a point in my professional development when I was at a university where I really did feel almost like giving up because I was told by someone in a position of authority that the field that I was engaged in, epidemiology, was not really a science.

And that as a woman if I wanted to be eligible for tenure, I would need to find a different discipline because I would have two strikes against me. I was very discouraged and very, very tearful, and then I got mad. And then I got energized, and I said, "No, that's not right; I'm a competent scientist; I'm going to be the best that I can be" (NewsHour, 2005).

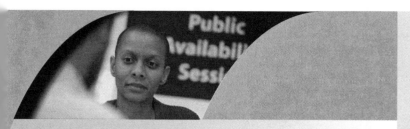

Discussion Questions

Consider the information provided in the chapter and the information described in the case study. Based on that information, discuss the following questions:

1. If you were in charge of implement a sweeping reorganization of the CDC, what management relationship behaviors would you used? Who would you target with these behaviors?

2. If you are a female, is there a need to act differently when you manage these relationships in an all-male leadership group?

3. If you are a male, is there a reason for a woman to act differently if she is managing a relationship with you?

4. Does the fact that Dr. Gerberding has expressed her own experience with discrimination make it more or less likely that she did not manage her relationship with the all-male management team well?

5. With such widespread dissatisfaction, how can Dr. Gerberding begin to manage relationships beyond the management team (using the LPI behaviors)?

6. Finally, what would be an effective communication plan at this point to address the discontent among the employees?

REFERENCES

Bombardieri M. Summers' remarks on women draw fire. *The Boston Globe*. January 17, 2005.

Catton W. Emile Who and the Division of What? *Sociological Perspectives*. 1985;28(3):251–280.

Charan R. The Collective Leadership of Boards. *Leader to Leader*. 2006;41: 38–40.

Fayol H. *General and Industrial Management*. London: Pitman; 1949.

Goleman D, Boyatzis R, McKee A. *Primal Leadership: Learning to Lead with Emotional Intelligence*. Boston: HBS Press; 2004.

Grabin, M. *You're the Time Study Man*. November 16, 2007. http://www .leanblog.org/2007/11/youre-time-study-man/.

Grint K. Leaders Are Trained, Not Born. *The Edge*. 2000(4).

Halberstam D. The Greatness That Cannot Be Taught. *Fast Company*. September 2004.

Harvard Business Review. On Breakthrough Leadership. *Primal Leadership: The Hidden Drive of Great Performance*. Cambridge, MA: Harvard Business School Press; 1979.

Hira N. Manage Us? Puh-leeze: Attracting the Twentysomething Worker. *Fortune*. May 28, 2007.

Kaiser Daily Health Policy Report—Kaiser Family Foundation. *Almost Two-Thirds of CDC Employees Oppose Reorganization Plan*. 2005. http://www .kaisernetwork.org/daily_reports/rep_index.cfm?hint=3&DR_ID=31665. Accessed August 4, 2008.

Kaiser Daily Health Policy Report—Kaiser Family Foundation. *Four Former NIOSH Directors Criticize CDC Reorganization Plan*. 2004. http://www .kaisernetwork.org/daily_reports/rep_index.cfm?DR_ID=24954. Accessed August 4, 2008.

Koontz H, O'Donnell C. *Principles of Management: An Analysis of Managerial Functions*. New York: McGraw-Hill Education; 1972.

Kouzes J, Posner B. *Leadership Practices Inventory (LPI): Facilitators Guide*. 2nd ed. San Francisco: Jossey-Bass and Pfeiffer; 1997.

Larson C., et al. *Colorado Healthy Communities Initiative: Ten Years Later*. Denver: Colorado Trust; 2002.

NewsHour. NewsHour with Jim Lehrer. *Special Report: Women and Science*. Available at: http://www.pbs.org/newshour/bb/science/jan-june05/harvard _02-22.html. Accessed August 4, 2008.

Rynders G. *Listening and Leadership: A Study of Their Relationship*. Sandy, UT: U.S. Fire Administration; 1999.

Preston P. Dealing with Difficult People. *Journal of Healthcare Management*. November/December 2005:367–370.

Turning Point. *Collaborative Leadership Learning Modules: A Comprehensive Series*. Seattle, WA: Robert Wood Johnson Foundation: University of Washington; 2006.

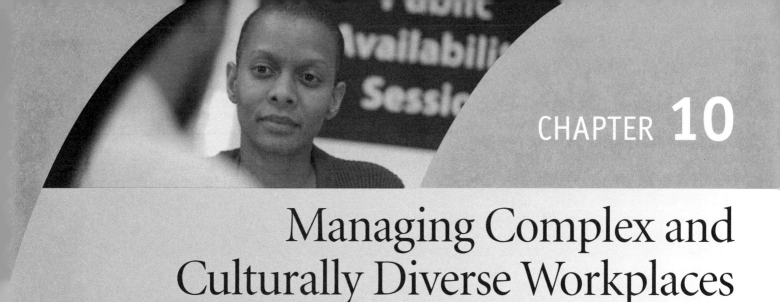

CHAPTER 10

Managing Complex and Culturally Diverse Workplaces

Sara Rosenbaum and Leonard H. Friedman

INTRODUCTION

This chapter explores the issue of managing diversity in the healthcare and public health workplace. The United States is a nation of extraordinary population diversity, a melting pot of multiple racial and ethnic subgroups and widely varying cultures. The expectation that workplaces, including public health and healthcare workplaces, reflect this diversity is a social one. Equally as important, the expectation of diversity is enshrined in multiple federal and state laws governing the conduct of public health agencies and healthcare enterprises, particularly those that (as is nearly universally the case) accept federal funds in the form of grants, contracts, and public health insurance payments.

Diversity transcends all locations; that is, whether the entity or organization is a small rural health department, a large academic health center, a nursing home, or a multisite community health center, both society and the legal system assume that health and healthcare entities will reflect the communities in which they operate. This expectation exists as a matter of established civil rights law. In recent years, this social and legal expectation of diversity has been increasingly grounded in the concept of healthcare quality, as health services research has documented the importance to overall healthcare quality improvement of focusing especially on those patient and community subpopulations at greatest risk for poor health outcomes and barriers to appropriate health care.

The theme of diversity appears throughout this text and serves as a platform and backdrop for many of the ideas and themes in this book. Healthcare corporate compliance is another aspect of diversity, which depends in part on adherence to civil rights requirements. Considerations related to legal liability, error reduction, and performance improvement also point toward a diverse healthcare workplace, as do the fulfillment of public health agency obligations to advance the core functions of public health: assessment, policy development, and assurance. So essential is workplace diversity to achieving quality and equality in health and health care that managing for diversity is now understood to be an essential function of public health and healthcare leadership.

LEARNING OBJECTIVES

After reading this chapter, the reader will be able to:

1. Define what is meant by workplace diversity.
2. Explain the multipronged rationale that underlies the goal of workplace diversity.
3. Understand the legal environment in which public health and healthcare managers operate, which creates a formal expectation of workplace diversity, not merely as an aim of high-quality management, but also as a matter of law.
4. Describe those management practices that are considered integral to attaining and maintaining a highly diverse workplace.

WORKPLACE DIVERSITY

Workplace Diversity Defined

Workplace diversity is a concept that extends well beyond an ability to show compliance with a host of federal and state laws that together require nondiscrimination in the workplace on the basis of race, ethnicity, primary language spoken, religion, disability, sex, or age. The essence of workplace diversity is its capacity to produce positive outcomes in relation to a host of performance measures; put another way, in a complex, globally oriented, and highly competitive world, workplace inclusiveness is viewed as an outcome in its own right, a result that is understood as essential to high performance, competitiveness, and success in corporate conduct and public management. A diverse workplace is one that respects and values differences among people and points of view and fosters an environment in which many views and perspectives can flourish as a management ideal (Society for Human Resources Management, 2008). Indeed, workplace diversity is considered so important that in *Grutter* v. *Bollinger*,[1] the landmark U.S. Supreme Court case that addressed the constitutionality of affirmative action as part of public higher education admissions programs, the record 44 *amicus curiae* (i.e., "friend of the court") briefs included briefs by leaders in industry and public service that stressed the importance of a diverse workforce, along with carefully crafted affirmative action efforts (Ward, 2007).

The Evidentiary Basis for Diversity in the Healthcare Workplace

This section explores the evidence base for healthcare workplace diversity, including diversity in both healthcare settings and in relation to public health practice.

There is substantial literature—much of it captured in two seminal reports by the Institute of Medicine (IOM)—that links both population health and healthcare quality to the existence of the diverse healthcare workforce that is essential to enabling diversity in the healthcare workplace.[2] As the IOM reports suggest, much of this literature comes from studies that focus on the issue of racial and ethnic diversity, but many of the points made in these studies reasonably can be presumed to carry over into other aspects of diversity, such as diversity on the basis of sex, gender orientation and identity, disability, age, and religious beliefs.

Racial and Ethnic Healthcare Workforce Diversity

In its report *Health Care's Compelling Interest: Ensuring Diversity in the Health-Care Workforce*, the IOM focused on institutional and policy barriers that impede efforts to achieve a more diverse healthcare workforce, noting the marked contrast between the rapid growth of racial and ethnic minority groups in the United States and their presence in the healthcare workforce. The IOM found a "several-fold" gap between the racial and ethnic composition of the population as a whole and the healthcare workforce population. For example, Hispanics comprise 12% of the population but only 2% of nurses; similarly, more than 12% of the population is African American, yet only 5% of all dentists are African American.[3]

The IOM concluded that a significant aspect of this serious minority healthcare workforce shortage can be found at the institutional level and with public policy impediments to the creation of a minority healthcare workforce. Where public policy is concerned, the IOM noted the reversal, by means of legislative referenda and court challenges, of longstanding efforts by educational institutions (particularly those undertaken by public colleges and universities) to achieve a more diverse healthcare workforce.[4] The impact of this reversal has been profound declines in student diversity, and the IOM stressed the importance of reversing this downward trend through strategies aimed at restoring and sustaining an institutional-level response capable of counteracting this deep shift in public policy. Specifically, the IOM made recommendations relating to recruitment and admission practices, the development of an educational "climate" for diversity, the use of institutional accreditation to student diversity and inclusion of diversity-related competency training as part of the health professions education process, and the creation of institutional-level financial incentives (through the use of health professions training funds and other sources of funding) to achieve greater diversity.

The IOM summarized the evidentiary basis on which its recommendations rested as follows:

> greater diversity among health professionals is associated with improved access to care for racial and ethnic minority patients, greater patient choice and satisfaction, and better patient-clinician communication. . . . Indirectly evidence suggests that greater diversity can improve the cultural competence of health professionals and health systems and that such improvements may be associated with better healthcare outcomes. In addition, greater diversity among health professionals has the potential to improve the clinical research enterprise and to lead to new developments and improvements in health care and how care is delivered.[5]

---

[1] *Grutter* v. *Bollinger*, 539 U.S. 306, 123 S. Ct. 2325 (2003).

[2] IOM, *Unequal Treatment: What Healthcare Providers Need to Know About Racial and Ethnic Disparities in Healthcare* (IOM, Washington, DC: Institute of Medicine, 2002); IOM, *Health Care's Compelling Interest: Ensuring Diversity in the Health-Care Workforce* (IOM, Washington, DC: Institute of Medicine, 2005).

---

[3] *Health Care's Compelling Interest*, 23–24.

[4] Id., 24.

[5] Id., 29.

In its review of the evidence, the IOM found that health-care workforce diversity tended to be associated with certain significant outcomes.

Access The first such outcome is access. The evidence suggests a measurable relationship between workforce diversity and healthcare access, particularly the documented barriers faced by minority populations as a result of language access. The IOM found, for example, that nearly one in five Spanish-speaking U.S. residents delayed or refused necessary care because of language barriers; similarly, nearly half of all Asian Americans and Pacific Islanders face barriers in securing necessary mental health services because of limited English proficiency.[6] While the IOM did not conclude that minority patients receive better health care when there is racial and ethnic concordance between caregivers and patients, it did find that greater workforce diversity does have an effect on access, as well as an overall effect on how healthcare entities generally respond to the needs of minority patients.[7] The evidence also shows that where the workforce includes greater numbers of racial and ethnic minority professionals, minority patients are more likely to make greater use of appropriate care, particularly ambulatory care for physical and mental health conditions that that are ambulatory care sensitive.[8]

Patient Choice and Satisfaction The IOM also found sufficient evidence to conclude that minority patients tend to seek care from health professionals who are members of their own racial or ethnic groups. Some of this care-seeking behavior may be the result of location: minority health professionals tend to practice in closer proximity to minority communities. Some of this tendency also can be traced to matters of language access, a fundamental aspect of healthcare quality. But there is also evidence that minority patients will choose providers who share their personal characteristics for reasons related to shared cultural experiences, greater use of shared decision-making approaches to care, world outlooks, and ability to achieve empathic communication, also key to quality of care.[9] Thus, where choice is available, patients will tend to choose in a racially concordant fashion. Put another way, in a highly competitive healthcare environment, assuring a diverse healthcare workforce offers a basic means of addressing issues of customer choice and satisfaction.

Healthcare Quality The IOM found that even controlling for health insurance coverage (minority populations are significantly more likely to lack appropriate coverage), patients who are members of racial and ethnic minority groups tend to receive health care of lower quality. Many of these findings rested on the findings contained in *Unequal Treatment*, the IOM's seminal study of race, ethnicity, and healthcare quality. Where healthcare quality is concerned, the evidence supports the conclusion that even when insured at the same level as white patients, minority patients tend to receive fewer clinical services and a lower quality of care even when they do have access. This basic conclusion spans a broad range of conditions, clinical services, and clinical settings. The IOM noted that "no direct link has been established as yet between diversity among health care clinicians and health outcomes for patients. . ." At the same time, the review concluded that "[h]ealth care processes and outcomes are influenced by cultural and linguistic barriers that minority clinicians are sometimes able to address" as a result of factors such as language concordance and the ability to "display better process of care behaviors with minority patients." The IOM concluded that minority providers may be able to achieve greater adherence to treatment plans as a result of language and cultural concordance, an intermediate outcome that "may affect patients' health outcomes, in that patient satisfaction is associated with greater patient compliance with treatment regiments, participation in treatment decisions, and use of preventive care services."[10]

Improvement in the Clinical Research Enterprise In the IOM's view, diversity in the healthcare workforce is also linked to the quality of research into racial and ethnic minority patient disparities in health and health care. The evidence suggests that minority scientists and researchers bring unique perspectives to the process of research, which in turn promotes research design approaches that are better able to identify underlying factors and causes associated with disparities. The presence of minority clinician/investigators also significantly improves the potential to recruit minority patients into clinical trials, a major goal of any healthcare institution with a major research component, such as an academic medical center or a teaching health center.

In summary, the goal of a diverse healthcare workplace rests on more than simply a strongly felt moral or ethical belief that the public health and healthcare systems should reflect the communities they serve. The IOM stresses the evidentiary basis for

[6]Id., 26.
[7]Id., 23–24.
[8]Id., 28–30.
[9]Id., 31–33.
[10]Id., 32–33.

healthcare workforce diversity: evidence of improved access to care; evidence of greater levels of patient satisfaction; evidence of improved healthcare utilization, leading to better health outcomes and the reduction of disparities in health and health care; and a more dynamic and high-performing research enterprise.

Diversity in the Public Health Workplace

The IOM report focuses in particular on diversity in the healthcare workforce. The same points can be made in the case of the public health workforce, where the issue of diversity is linked less to the clinical process of care and individual patient outcomes and more to the successful achievement of the core functions of public health. Three core functions characterize the public health enterprise: assessment, assurance, and policy development. A diverse public health workforce, along with a public health work environment that emphasizes and advances diversity, is essential to the performance of any of these three functions. The case for diversity in public health practice and workplaces rests on the same considerations as those that the IOM found with respect to clinical workforce diversity—namely, the ways in which diversity affects the ability of healthcare professionals to effectively communicate with patients and to bring to the healthcare enterprise knowledge and insights critical to healthcare quality.

In the area of public health, it is difficult to imagine how the challenges of assessment, policy development, and assurance can be effectively accomplished in the absence of a diverse workforce and diversity in the workplace. The core public health function of assessment means, of course, assessing patterns of subpopulation health within larger communities and being able to understand and take into account the factors that might help explain the underlying causes of health disparities or health risk factors. The official literature on population health disparities on the basis of race, ethnicity, income and other factors is vast.[11] Much of the public health assessment function has as its purpose understanding these disparity patterns and, through policy development and assurance, effectively responding to them.

Without cultural competence and a diverse workforce, the chances rise that population health assessments will miss key factors that contribute to racial and ethnic disparities in death and disability related to manmade or naturally occurring environmental disasters;[12] infant mortality;[13] or the incidence

and burden of chronic diseases such as diabetes, cardiovascular disease, or serious depression.[14] For the same reasons, the absence of cultural competence makes it far more difficult to formulate effective policies to reduce population health disparities. Similarly, it becomes far more difficult to perform the function of ensuring access to services and interventions that can improve health, or to assess the effects of interventions aimed at improving health and reducing disparities. For this reason, initiatives aimed at improving the performance of public health agencies have emphasized a more diverse public health workforce and workplace diversity as central goals.[15]

The Legal Basis of Healthcare Workforce Diversity

This section explores the legal basis of health workforce diversity and summarizes the various bodies of law that come into play where diversity is concerned.

The definition of diversity, noted earlier in this chapter, extends well beyond the obligations of virtually all healthcare entities and public health agencies to ensure nondiscrimination against certain historically underrepresented population groups, such as members of racial and ethnic minority populations, persons with disabilities, older persons, or women. Most of the workplace diversity challenges that effective public health managers face stem from cultural, social, and financial considerations related to both care for individual patients and broader community benefit. In other words, regardless of legal requirements, it is in the social and economic interest of a healthcare entity, and part of the basic community obligation of a public health agency, to ensure high performance for patients and communities.

For example, a hospital needs to be able to capably and sensitively respond to the needs of patients with HIV/AIDS, which may include many gay men with the condition. Beyond the need for clinical competence in caring for individual gay men who are patients, the hospital may be located in a service area that encompasses a sizable gay, lesbian, bisexual, and transgender community. In this case, the hospital's considerations are more than the quality of its patient care for individual patients; the facility has a major economic interest in being

[11]U.S. Department of Health and Human Services, Healthy People 2010; NCHS, Health, United States (2007).

[12]Eric Klinenberg, *Heatwave: A Social Autopsy of Disaster in Chicago,* University of Chicago Press, 2002.

[13]IOM, Preventing Low Birthweight. http://www.nap.edu/openbook.php?record_id=512&page=R1 , accessed February 18, 2010.

[14]NCHS, Fast Stats, http://www.cdc.gov/nchs/fastats/black_health.htm, accessed August 9, 2008.

[15]Elizabeth M. Krause, Making the Case for Workforce Diversity in Public Health, http://www.cdphe.state.co.us/ohd/reportsandarticles/making-casearticle.pdf, accessed August 9, 2008; Daniel M. Harper, A Diverse Environmental Public Health Workforce to Meet the Diverse Environmental Health Challenges of the 21st Century http://www.cdc.gov/nceh/ehs/Docs/JEH/2007/Jan-Feb_2007_Harper.pdf, accessed August 9, 2009; Dennis Mitchell and Shanna Lassiter, Addressing Health Care Disparities and Increasing Workforce Diversity: The Next Step for the Dental, Medical, and Public Health Professions, *AJPH* 96:12 (Oct 31, 2006).

viewed as a high-quality source of care for the community and the public and private health insurers and group health benefit plans that insure the members of the community and pay the bills. Thus, whether or not there exist specific human rights or civil rights laws in a particular state or locality that prohibit discrimination based on sexual orientation or gender status, it is in the interest of the hospital to achieve workplace diversity where patient treatment is concerned. Simply stated, as stressed in the corporate *amicus* briefs in *Grutter* v. *Bollinger*, workplace diversity is good for business. Similarly, it is in the direct interest of a public health agency, with community assessment and assurance responsibilities, to achieve workplace diversity in the context of sexual orientation and gender status because of the unique issues that arise in being able to competently identify health conditions and design appropriate remedies.

As a result of these issues and developments, there now exists a considerable body of law that addresses diversity in the context of nondiscrimination. The laws that govern nondiscrimination in the workplace are complex; at the same time, they can be summarized as follows:

1. The law prohibits intentional discrimination against certain protected population subgroups.
2. The law does not compel any particular diversity outcome, only that discrimination not be the intended or *de facto* (effective) result of workplace practices.
3. The law prohibits the use of hard quotas to achieve workplace diversity; at the same time however, the law favors the use of well-designed and narrowly tailored practices in recruitment, workplace employment, and the conditions of employment, which can help promote a diverse workplace that is reflective of the community it serves.

Categories of Nondiscrimination Laws: Legally Protected Populations

It is impossible in so brief a space to do more than scratch the surface of laws that regulate workplace practices, including nondiscrimination. A full discussion of applicable law would span both federal and state legislation and would encompass both public laws (e.g., constitutions and statutes) as well as legally enforceable obligations created by contracts between parties. The discussion that follows is intended to provide a roadmap for understanding the legal dimensions of workplace diversity.

Federal and State Statutes and Constitutions

Federal and state laws recognize certain discrete subpopulations as entitled to protection against discrimination. In some cases, these laws have a specific basis in the Constitution (such

as federal laws prohibiting discrimination on the basis of race). In other cases, lawmakers have enacted specific protections (extending beyond the reach of constitutional guarantees of equal protection against discrimination by governmental entities) because of clear evidence of past and ongoing discrimination (such as laws prohibiting discrimination on the basis of disability).[16] For these legally protected populations, laws against discrimination, whether based directly in the Constitution or in statute, reach workplace discrimination, spanning all phases of work, from recruitment to compensation (including noncash wages and employee benefits such as health and disability benefits) and other conditions of employment (i.e., the workplace environment).

Federal laws extend legal protection against discrimination to certain specific groups: qualified persons with disabilities; individuals based on race, national origin, skin color, sex, or religion; and older workers.[17] In addition, state laws may recognize certain additional populations as deserving legal protection; state laws vary significantly depending on the state. For example, certain states have laws that prohibit employment discrimination on the basis of sexual orientation or gender identity.[18] Other states may extend specific protections for persons with certain conditions such as HIV/AIDS. Thus, an essential step in creating and maintaining a healthcare corporate compliance plan (discussed later) is ascertaining the specific laws of the state in which the business operates.

Federal Laws Prohibiting Workplace Discrimination and Promoting Diversity: Civil Rights Laws

A series of federal civil rights laws prohibit workplace discrimination. The most prominent of these laws are Title VII of the 1964 Civil Rights Act (Title VII), the Age Discrimination in Employment Act (ADEA), and the Americans with Disabilities Act (ADA).

Title VII: Discrimination on the Basis of Race, Skin Color, Religion, Sex, and National Origin Title VII of the Civil Rights Act of 1964,[19] is the nation's most sweeping federal civil rights law related to discrimination in employment. The law,

[16]Rand Rosenblatt, Sylvia Law, and Sara Rosenbaum, *Law and the American Health Care System* (New York: Foundation Press, 1997) (2001–2002 Supplement).

[17]See a full description of protected persons at the website of the Equal Employment Opportunity Commission, http://www.eeoc.gov/abouteeo/overview_laws.html, accessed August 9, 2008.

[18]An excellent resource for identifying state laws on matters of sexual orientation or gender identity can be found at the LAMBDA Legal Defense and Education Fund. See "In Your State," http://www.lambdalegal.org/our-work/states/new-york.html, accessed August 9, 2008.

[19]42 U.S.C. §2000e.

part of the landmark Civil Rights Act of 1964, protects individuals from discrimination based on their race, national origin, skin color, sex, or religion. Title VII reaches both public and private employers employing 15 or more persons on a full-time basis (defined as 20 or more weeks annually). (Many states have parallel laws that reach small employers.) Title VII does not reach federal employees nor does it cover state and local employees subject to civil service requirements; separate legal protections, that may or may not be as broad as Title VII, apply to these groups of employees.[20] In sum, Title VII has, as its fundamental purpose, the protection of persons working for medium and large private employers. Thus, for example, a 10-person physician practice might not be covered by Title VII but might be subject to state anti-discrimination or human rights laws.

The concept of discrimination based on religion under Title VII reaches all aspects of religious observance or practice,[21] while discrimination based on sex reaches discrimination involving pregnancy and childbirth.[22]

Title VII sets out a detailed range of prohibited practices, employment practices that are considered exempt from the prohibitions of the statute, and specific defenses to claims of discrimination. Specifically, the Act provides that it is unlawful

> (1) to fail or refuse to hire or to discharge any individual, or otherwise to discriminate against any individual with respect to . . . compensation, terms, conditions, or privileges of employment, because of such individual's race, color, religion, sex, or national origin; or
>
> (2) to limit, segregate, or classify his employees or applicants for employment in any way which would deprive or tend to deprive any individual of employment opportunities or otherwise adversely affect his status as an employee, because of such individual's race, color, religion, sex, or national origin.
>
> (b) . . . for an employment agency to fail or refuse to refer for employment, or otherwise to discriminate against, any individual because of his race, color, religion, sex, or national origin, or to classify or refer for employment any individual on the basis of his race, color, religion, sex, or national origin.

> (c) . . . for a labor organization (1) to exclude or to expel from its membership, or otherwise to discriminate against, any individual because of his race, color, religion, sex, or national origin; (2) to limit, segregate, or classify its membership or applicants for membership, or to classify or fail or refuse to refer for employment any individual, in any way which would deprive or tend to deprive any individual of employment opportunities, or would limit such employment opportunities or otherwise adversely affect his status as an employee or as an applicant for employment, because of such individual's race, color, religion, sex, or national origin; . . .
>
> (d) . . . for any employer, labor organization, or joint labor–management committee controlling apprenticeship or other training or retraining, including on-the-job training programs to discriminate against any individual because of his race, color, religion, sex, or national origin in admission to, or employment in, any program . . . [23]

Title VII thus sweeps broadly, reaching hiring, apprenticeships, and on-the-job training programs, all aspects of compensation and workplace environment matters such as harassment. Title VII reaches union conduct and labor management committees and extends to both direct discrimination as well as practices that would "tend to" cause discrimination.

Furthermore, the concept of "because of" (as in refusing to hire or promote or firing a person *because of* race, sex, skin color, national origin, or religion) does not depend on a showing of intentional discrimination. Title VII can be violated if it can be shown that the use of employment practices, selection and testing methods, work requirements, disciplinary practices, or other employment practices has a disparate impact on one or more protected groups. Thus, in reviewing the legality of specific employer practices, federal regulators and courts can consider both the disparate treatment and disparate impact of specified conduct. What differentiates the two types of conduct is an employer's intent. Cases that are classified as "disparate treatment" cases involve discriminatory employment decisions that are motivated by or based on a protected characteristic of an individual, such as race, sex, or national origin. By contrast, employment practices that would be viewed as having a discriminatory impact would involve the application of a "facially neutral" policy or practice that has an unintended

---

[20]42 U.S.C. §2000e(f).

[21]42 U.S.C. §2000e(j).

[22]42 U.S.C. §2000e(k).

[23]42 U.S.C. §2000e-2.

negative consequence on a particular protected group.[24] For this reason, disparate impact conduct focuses on "practices that are fair in form, but discriminatory in operation."[25]

Title VII is administered by the Equal Employment Opportunity Commission (EEOC).[26] The EEOC is charged with Title VII enforcement and in furtherance of this power, Title VII §709(c) requires every covered employer to make, keep, and preserve records that are "relevant to the determinations of whether unlawful employment practices have been or are being committed."[27] Thus, Title VII contains an employer-focused record-keeping provision that ensures that relevant data on employee characteristics is collected and maintained. These EEOC requirements have been specifically sanctioned by the U.S. Supreme Court.[28]

Notwithstanding its broad sweep, Title VII contains significant limitations in addition to those already noted. First, the burden of proof is on a plaintiff to show discrimination, whether *de facto* or intentional, and proving a discrimination case, in particular one that relates to facially neutral practices, can be exceedingly difficult. Second, Title VII creates a "business necessity" affirmative defense that permits an employer to attempt to demonstrate that a particular facially neutral practice "is a bona fide occupational qualification reasonably necessary to the normal operation of that particular business or enterprise. . ."[29] Thus, for example, where certain types of healthcare occupations require a minimum level of reading comprehension skills or the ability to work certain hours or days of the week, even where the practice disproportionately affects certain groups of employees, an employer may be able to show the reasonable business necessity of the practice. At the same time, a business necessity defense, to succeed, must be shown to involve a business need that is reasonable and that is not capable of being satisfied in an alternative approach.

The Age Discrimination in Employment Act (ADEA) Enacted in 1967, the ADEA was the result of congressional concern regarding evidence of forced retirement, job displacement, long-term unemployment, and hiring and promotion preferences that favor younger workers. As with Title VII, the ADEA reaches both intentional and *de facto* discrimination and is de-

signed to protect workers 40 years of age or older.[30] The workplace practice prohibitions under the ADEA are highly similar to those found under Title VII; thus, it is unlawful for covered entities (firms employing 20 or more persons)

> (1) to fail or refuse to hire or to discharge any individual or otherwise discriminate against any individual with respect to his compensation, terms, conditions, or privileges of employment, because of such individual's age; [or]
>
> (2) to limit, segregate, or classify his employees in any way which would deprive or tend to deprive any individual of employment opportunities or otherwise adversely affect his status as an employee, because of such individual's age . . .[31]

As is the case with Title VII, covered employers that can show a reasonable business need or a bona fide occupational qualification related to age have an affirmative defense against liability under the ADEA.[32] Thus, for example, where an employer can show that a maximum age requirement is legitimately related to a reasonable business need, the practice would be permissible. Similarly, employers can vary retiree health benefits by age, granting full benefits to retirees under age 65, while limiting or excluding benefits for retirees who have reached Medicare eligibility.

Discrimination Based on Disability Title I of the Americans with Disabilities Act (ADA),[33] like the ADEA and Title VII, prohibits discrimination based on disability, whether intentional or *de facto*, unless an employer can demonstrate business need. Firms employing 15 or more full-time workers are covered. As with Title VII or the ADEA, many states provide additional protections covering small firms.

In order to fall within the ADA's protections, an individual must be considered "a qualified person with a disability." As a result of a series of U.S. Supreme Court decisions over the past decade, the concept of who is a qualified person with a disability has been considerably narrowed in an employment context. Under the ADA, the term disability means

> (A) a physical or mental impairment that substantially limits one or more of the major life activities of such individual; (B) a record of such an

---

[24] 42 U.S.C. §2000e(k)(i)(A).

[25] *Griggs* v. *Duke Power Co.*, 401 U.S. 424, (1971) at 431.

[26] 42 U.S.C. §2000e-4.

[27] 42 U.S.C. §2000e-9(c).

[28] *U.S.* v. *New Hampshire*, 539 F.2d 277 (C.A.N.H. 1976) at 280, quoting *Griggs* v. *Duke Power Co.*, 401 U.S. 424, 429-30 (1971).

[29] 42 U.S.C. §2000e-2(e).

[30] 29 U.S.C. §630.

[31] 29 U.S.C. §623.

[32] 29 U.S.C. §623(f).

[33] 42 U.S.C. §12111 et. seq.

impairment; or (C) being regarded as having such an impairment.[34]

Federal regulations implementing the ADA set forth an elaborate listing of impairments. But simply having one of the listed impairments is not sufficient to trigger ADA protections. In addition to having an impairment within the meaning of the law, a person must be "qualified"; that is, the individual must be

> an individual with a disability who, *with or without reasonable accommodation, can perform the essential functions* of the employment position that such individual holds or desires. For the purposes of this subchapter, consideration shall be given to the employer's judgment as to what functions of a job are essential, and if an employer has prepared a written description before advertising or interviewing applicants for the job, this description shall be considered evidence of the essential functions of the job.[35] [emphasis added]

It becomes evident from this statutory excerpt that the ADA vests considerable discretion in employers to determine essential job elements, particularly where job requirements are specified during the recruitment process. To trigger protection under the ADA, the individual must be able to demonstrate his or her ability to perform the essential functions of a job without regard to reasonable accommodation. In other words, if a job involves the ability to do data entry, then an individual with paraplegia could demonstrate that she is able to perform data entry regardless of whether the workspace is modified to permit the use of a wheelchair. If on the other hand, the job, in the opinion of the employer, requires perfect sight, an individual without perfect sight (even if the individual can prove perfect sight with the aid of corrective lenses) is not considered a qualified person with a disability.[36]

As with the ADEA or Title VII, employers are given certain defenses. In the context of the ADA, the most important defense is the "fundamental alteration" defense. That is, employers can show that an accommodation sought by a qualified individual with a disability is not reasonable but in fact is a fundamental alteration requiring an essential change in the nature of the activity or thing to be modified. Federal guidelines provide examples of reasonable modifications, clarifying that alterations such as ramps, grab bars, telecommunication devices, and other workplace adaptations are not considered fundamental.

In summary, despite their evident limitations, federal civil rights laws play an enormous role in the work environment. Perhaps their most important role is as formal statements that codify in law the national aim of inclusiveness and diversity. Put another way, while Title VII, the ADEA, and the ADA have clear limitations that tend to somewhat lessen the opening sweep and scope of their nondiscrimination standards, their very existence establishes a formal expectation of diversity, one that healthcare employers, like other employers, are expected to attain. Penalties for violation of these laws may be fines and other financial sanctions, but more important may be the publicity that comes with a violation.

Laws Compelling Diversity as a Condition of Federal Funding: Title VI Standards Governing Services for Persons with Limited English Proficiency (LEP)

Beyond federal civil rights laws, various federal programs that provide funding, whether in the form of grants or insurance payments, may contain specific conditions that create diversity obligations. For example, virtually all U.S. hospitals participate in Medicare and Medicaid, and thousands receive funding under various federal programs administered by the Centers for Disease Control and Prevention, the National Institutes of Health, and other federal health agencies. Participation in these programs makes hospitals (along with other healthcare providers)[37] "federally assisted entities" and as such, obligated to comply with Title VI of the 1964 Civil Rights Act. A companion to Title VII, Title VI prohibits both intentional and *de facto* discrimination and has been interpreted to prohibit discrimination on the basis of primary language spoken.

In 2000, the U.S. Department of Health and Human Services (HHS) promulgated landmark federal guidelines that spell out in detailed fashion the obligation of federally assisted entities to make their services language accessible.[38] This requirement has had a profound impact on workplace diversity in health care: it has propelled forward the concept of language access in health care, requiring covered healthcare entities to be able to communicate with patients in both oral and written form. In addition to written materials and technology adop-

---

[34]42 U.S.C. §12101 et. seq.

[35]42 U.S.C. §12111(8).

[36]*Law and the American Health Care System*. See *Sutton* v *United Airlines*. 527 U.S. 471, 119 S. Ct. 2139 (1999).

[37]Physicians who participate only in Medicare Part B on a fee-for-service basis (i.e., not as part of a Medicare Advantage provider network) are not considered federally assisted.

[38]U.S. Department of Health and Human Services, Limited English Proficiency, http://www.hhs.gov/ocr/lep/, accessed August 9, 2008.

tion, the Limited English Proficiency (LEP) Guidelines require the presence of formal interpreter services in larger facilities.

The LEP guidelines take a corporate compliance approach to implementation and enforcement. That is, covered entities are expected to carefully assess their services and the needs of their service areas and to then develop and vet a detailed plan for compliance that articulates goals, services, and the means by which the covered entity will engage in ongoing efforts to measure compliance with its standards.

Contractual Expectations and Duties In addition to public laws, workplace diversity may be a contractual obligation. For example, an employer group health plan administrator may require that hospitals that participate in its network demonstrate an ability to assist members with limited English proficiency. In this case, a hospital or physician who treats only privately insured patients, and that would be considered otherwise exempt from Title VI, may find that it has a contractual obligation to make its services accessible, an obligation that carries workplace diversity obligations.

Similarly, accreditation standards may specifically identify workplace diversity as an industry standard. As the IOM report discussed earlier in this chapter suggests, in recent years, accrediting bodies, for reasons of quality improvement and disparities reduction, have increasingly paid attention to the question of workplace diversity. Failure to have a diversity plan, to provide services and supports essential to diversity, and to attract and maintain a diverse workforce may all implicate ongoing accreditation.

Managing for Workplace Diversity

The prior sections and discussion have clearly shown that there is a large and respected body of public laws and contractual standards that require workplace diversity, ensuring that diversity-creating practices and policies in hiring and other employment practices become a matter of corporate compliance. As a result, corporate compliance plans can be expected to address the steps that a healthcare provider will take to achieve workforce diversity and to ensure the accessibility and quality of its care for the community it serves.

But for the reasons discussed in this chapter, diversity has a rationale that extends well beyond legal compliance. Diversity is an essential business practice in the case of healthcare providers, and it is central to the ability of public health agencies to perform the core functions of assessment, assurance, and policy development. Thus, successful management entails striving for diversity. Adherence to the legal requirements associated with diversity represents a necessary but not sufficient condition for public health organizations. The proactive

and insightful public health leader will make diversity one of the core values upon which his or her organization functions. Towards that end, four diversity-centric business strategies are recommended that will help effectively meet the needs of the community:

1. *Think broadly about diversity.* While the law requires public health leaders to comply with diversity regulations around race, gender, and age, these should only be the starting points. Are there other measures of diversity that might be included? Broad-based diversity allows the organization the opportunity to bring different perspectives, points of view, ways of thinking, and experiences to address issues and challenges in ways that are unavailable to organizations where diversity is not present. As there is not just one way to manage, there are many different ways to enhance diversity within a public health organization.

2. *Reflect the diversity of the population.* This idea was discussed earlier in this chapter but bears repeating. The makeup of the staff of the public health organization should reflect the makeup of the population it serves. Beyond the staff and clients looking alike is the great value when similar cultural values are shared. Nowhere in the law is cultural diversity required, but in order to be truly effective, the staff of the public health organization needs to understand (and share) the norms, beliefs, and values of the population they serve.

3. *Better meet the needs of clients.* Making population-based public health services available does not mean that those services will necessarily be used by those for whom the greatest need exists. Ensuring that needed services are available is only half of the equation. If these services are not used, then what is the point? Clients will use services if a history of trust, empathy, and goodwill has been established. Developing these attributes is never easy but is facilitated when staff mirrors the persons they serve.

4. *Enhance organizational performance.* This book has emphasized the need to think about public health management from a business perspective. This might appear to be antithetical to persons with a traditional public health background, but in an environment with shrinking revenues, an apathetic public, and increasing skepticism from elected officials, it is more important than ever to demonstrate the value of your organization to the communities you serve. Enhanced organizational performance around measurable goals is one crucial way to build support for your work and help

buffer your operations from what might be capricious and arbitrary budget reductions. Organizational diversity is one important tool by which you can build improved performance. Hiring a (broadly) diverse workforce helps allow the public health leader to better detect strong and weak signals in the environment, be able to create meaningful organizational change, and provide the breadth of services most needed by the community being served.

CONCLUSION

Strong public health management and good business practice suggests that the wise public health leader will continuously strive to create as diverse a workplace as possible. Diversity in public health organizations is a matter of both legal necessity and business imperative. Overriding either of these practices is the IOM report that draws our attention to the congruence between workplace diversity and our ability to meet the needs of the communities we serve. We have seen that there are a number of federal laws that speak clearly to the need for public health leaders to comply with regulations around nondiscrimination in hiring and promotion. Diversity should not be limited to just ethnicity, age, physical ability, or gender, and should be thought of very broadly. A public health workplace that embraces diversity of thought and opinion will allow the organization to make better decisions and be more resilient in the face of change and uncertainty in what is already a very complex environment.

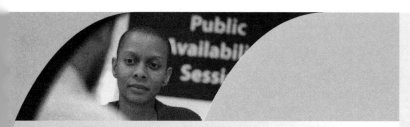

Discussion Questions

1. What seem to be the characteristics of a truly diverse public health organization?

2. One of the most controversial diversity laws is the Americans with Disabilities Act (ADA). What is it about this law that seems to be so troublesome, and why do so many employers complain so loudly about the law?

3. Briefly outline how you might recommend your public health organization comply with the EEOC and ADEA requirements.

4. Why do communities and/or healthcare organizations fear diversity?

5. What do communities do to increase awareness of diversity?

6. Provide a single-page memo to the administrator of your organization, making the business case for significantly enhanced diversity in your workplace. How are you going to do this in a budget-neutral manner?

CITATIONS

Society for Human Resource Management, "Diversity Defined in Less Than One Third of Workplaces," http://www.shrm.org/press_published/1CMS_024745.asp#P-4_0, accessed August 8, 2008.

Stephanie W. Friends of the Court are Friends of Mine, *ABA Journal* (November 2007), http://abajournal.com/magazine/friends_of_the_court_are_friends_of_mine/, accessed August 8, 2008.

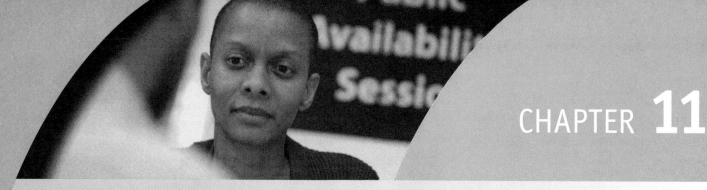

CHAPTER 11

Fundraising, Grant Writing, Budgeting, and Project Management

Robert E. Burke and Pam Larmee

INTRODUCTION

In today's business and not-for-profit worlds, financial operations of public health agencies and programs are complex and often competitive. It is imperative that public health and health services leaders and managers understand the importance of fundraising, grant writing, budgeting, and project management to the financial success and growth of their organizations. Over the past years, we have learned that the success of the public health organization is tied to success of obtaining external funding. In most circumstances, the financial allocations provided by government and/or private agencies do not cover all the expenses for most public health programs. In addition to other managerial skills that have been described in previous chapters, the manager must also be a fundraiser. For many managers this is a new role. It is also a time-consuming and taxing task because as competition for dollars grows ever tighter, it is truly a situation of the survival of the fittest.

In the 21st century, public health managers and leaders must be prepared to:

Secure a diverse base of funding sources.
Create a transparent budget.
Implement strategic financial management plans.

These basic building blocks create a strong organization that has the resources it needs to move its business and mission forward.

This chapter's goal is to create an understanding of the many facets of fundraising as well as to build awareness about the interdependence of transparent budgeting, strategic financial management, and fundraising.

LEARNING OBJECTIVES

After reading this chapter, the reader will be able to:

1. Identify a variety of fundraising and nonbusiness revenue sources.
2. Define fundraising revenue types.
3. Understand philanthropic trends.
4. Describe overviews of federal/state agency contract and grant proposals, foundation/corporate foundation proposals, and individual/family proposals.
5. Understand fundraising staffing patterns.
6. Discuss current ethical issues in fundraising.
7. Describe the importance of transparent budgets and project management to fundraising.
8. Understand how to set organizational fundraising strategy.

PRINCIPLES OF HEALTHCARE PHILANTHROPY

A Diverse Base of Funding Sources

Public health and health services organizations, the vast majority of which are not-for-profits, often run on very tight financial allocations and margins. As a result, they must be attentive and open to all possible funding sources outside of business revenues.[1] These sources range from membership dues to outright gifts. **Figure 11-1** graphically depicts what may be included as a financial source. This funding source diagram represents two interdependent measures: transactional versus

---

[1] *Business revenues* are the sources of the agency's or program's usual and customary financial support or money. For some agencies, it may be a direct allocation of a state budget; for others, it may be an allocation from an agency within a state or regional office or program.

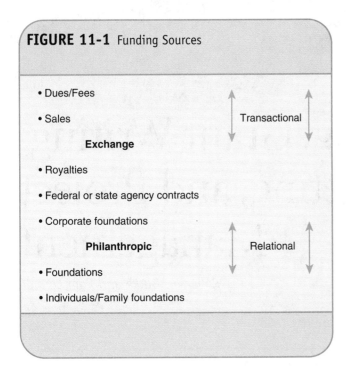

FIGURE 11-1 Funding Sources

- Dues/Fees
- Sales

Transactional

Exchange

- Royalties
- Federal or state agency contracts
- Corporate foundations

Philanthropic

Relational

- Foundations
- Individuals/Family foundations

relational and exchange versus philanthropic. As transactional relationships become relational opportunities, the funding relationship between them moves from exchange to philanthropic. Excluding business revenues, organizational leaders and managers should understand that while it takes less time and fewer resources to invest in transactional/exchange opportunities, the financial reward curve is significantly greater within in a relational/philanthropic relationship.

While transactional opportunities offer vital financial resources to an organization, they are often limited in size, both in terms of potential audience as well as duration, because exchange transactions are not often viewed by the donor as significant investments in an organization. On the other hand, relational fundraising opportunities are growth sectors for an organization's resource base. These funding relationships are based on the power of involvement, mission, and altruism, with their largest successes or payoffs coming over time as relationships grow and evolve. And while organizations do need a combination of exchange and philanthropic funding opportunities, because there are many different entry points for revenue generation, investing in relationships has a more significant upside. As philanthropic relationships develop, four tenets should guide organizational behavior:

1. Potential funders do not "owe" any organization financial support. While it may be a mutually beneficial relationship, it is one defined by asking and receiving.

2. Each organization is its own best advocate. Requests for funds must be defined by strong messages, measurable outcomes, and a sense of urgency in order to create the most compelling opportunity for a potential funder to say "yes" to a proposal.

3. Gifts are made to an organization for the purpose requested. Gifts are not made to an individual representing the organization. Requests are not personal; they are on behalf of an organization.

4. Funding is highly competitive. It is not automatic, and prioritizing fundraising is critical to ensuring that an organization has the resources it needs to carry out its mission.

Revenue Types

All of the funding sources previously mentioned result in operational resources for public health and health services organizations. With revenue that is considered philanthropic, or the result of fundraising, there are three general categories, all of which have different impacts on an organization's bottom line:

- *Unrestricted revenue:* gifts made to an organization to support general work and capacity. These gifts can be used to support any part of the organization's work, including operations/bottom-line needs, and are generally expended on an annual basis.
- *Restricted revenue:* gifts made to an organization to support specific projects and programs. These gifts can only be used for the stated purposes for which they are accepted and are generally expended on an annual basis.
- *Endowment:* gifts made to an organization to support specific projects and programs for which the principal of the gift is preserved in perpetuity and annually only a percentage of interest earned is used to support the specific project or program.

Unrestricted contributions are the most difficult to fundraise. In today's financial climate, donors are seeking greater organizational accountability, and they perceive that they better understand exactly how restricted gifts will be utilized. As a result, more and more donors are shifting from making unrestricted gifts in favor of making gifts that have some restrictions on them. For example, today's donor may have a greater interest in making a gift to support a restricted program area (outreach, research, field work, etc.), rather than a general gift to support an organization. However, even given this trend, organizations cannot lose sight that operational/unrestricted fundraising is not optional, but rather a critical financial component. These unrestricted gifts allow organizations the flexibility to use contributions in the best possible way, whether for programs or administrative costs.

Philanthropic Trends

As public health and health services organizations consider which funding sources they want to pursue and in what areas they have the greatest chances of success, leaders need to consider the broad picture of philanthropy in the United States. One tool is *Giving USA*, a publication of Giving USA Foundation™, researched and written by the Center on Philanthropy at Indiana University, published annually. For more than 50 years, this report has tracked, year to year, philanthropic trends that are important for organizations to monitor and understand as they develop and refine their own philanthropic plans.

In 2007, overall giving to charities in the United States totaled more than $306 billion—an increase of 1% after inflation adjustment from 2006. Organizations should note from where the philanthropic dollars originated (note that numbers are rounded and may not equal 100%):

- Individuals gave 75% of the total. Although the majority of gifts are in the $100 range, there are still thousands of much larger gifts.
- Foundations gave 13% of the total.
- Bequests from individuals generated 8% of the total.
- Corporations/corporate foundations gave 5% of the total (Hrywna, 2008).

In creating an effective philanthropic matrix for an organization, health services and public health leaders should bear in mind that, in aggregate, individuals give close to 85% of the total philanthropic dollars, while corporations, corporate foundations, and foundations give a little more than 15% of the total. Financially successful organizations create varied, unique philanthropy roadmaps that include both short- and long-term payoffs.

To better understand the gifts given by individuals, Del Martin, chair of Giving USA Foundation™, related that "some 51 percent of individual giving comes from the 10 percent of households in the highest income groups and slightly less coming from the 90 percent with income less than $100,000. "While higher-income families are major donors to many important institutions, ordinary-income donors are vital, too, for the health of the nonprofit sector in this country" (*Giving USA Shows Bequests*, 2008).

Fundraising Basics

As an organization increases its philanthropy, health services and public health organizational leaders should create a template to help:

- Determine which funding sources are better organizational matches than others.
- Understand basic fundraising approaches.
- Anticipate potential bottom-line impacts.

There are three large subsets of philanthropic resources: federal/state agency contracts and grants, foundation/corporate foundation grants, and gifts from individuals/families.

Federal and State Agency Contract and Grant Proposal Overview

Federal and state contracts and grants represent the "gray area" between exchange and philanthropic relationships because they contain aspects of both funding arenas. Indeed, fund-seekers must pay close attention to both parts of the funding equation to be successful. For example, an organization that is applying for government funding must strictly adhere to all of the written rules concerning its application. Over time, however, it is sometimes possible that an organization may enjoy "previous funder" status, which enables it to advance more readily through the early stages of the funding process. This elevated status is a result of following the guidelines exactly and maximizing the funder relationship over time by delivering timely results in the manner proposed.

There are important distinctions between a grant and a contract. *Grants* are legal agreements to execute projects within broad limits that allow for consultation between parties before and during the process. In most cases, if the grant outcomes are not as predicted, there are no legal ramifications as long as the efforts to achieve the results are documented. *Contracts,* on the other hand, are legal agreements to achieve an outcome or deliver a product according to specifications. Once the request for contract proposals (RFP) has been released, there is no discussion between the contract seeker and the contracting agency. Ultimately, there are often legal ramifications if the goods or services are not produced (Burke, 2008).

Grant and contract proposals generally fall into two categories: technical and business. *Technical proposals* are most successful when there is clear language describing the statement of the problem, the technical approach being put forward, the tasking divisions, the management plan, and the organization's "past performance" record. They also contain supporting documentation including résumés and blurbs, corporate capabilities, endorsements, and teaming agreements as well as exhibits such as organizational charts, labor loading diagrams, skills matrixes, task lists, deliverables, and timelines. Often, technical proposals are very prescriptive, and an organization will be best served by directly adhering to the guidelines (Burke, 2008).

Business proposals are slightly less formulaic and are often written with a more persuasive tone than technical proposals. Business proposals describe a compelling case statement, the technical approach to be utilized, a project timeline, the expected outcomes, an "urgency" message, a basic strategic plan, a record of past performance, and a donor appeal. These components are supported with résumés, additional documentation, relevant reference materials, and partnership documentation/endorsement (Burke, 2008).

These two sections, the technical proposal and the business proposal are scored by the funding agency. Some agencies use internal staff to score proposals, while others use study panels of experts or even another contractor. Depending on how the agency does its work, the agency will typically choose two or three proposals and ask additional questions or ask for an oral presentation that will be considered the bidder's "best and final offer." For example, in many competitive proposals, the agency decides on a range of acceptable scores for the technical proposal. Those technical proposals that met the score will be considered acceptable to the agency and are then all considered to be on an equal playing field. The pricing or business proposal is opened and, again typically, the proposal with the lowest cost wins the contract. Before writing a proposal, we strongly advise reading all the instructions and all the proposal criteria in detail. Many a proposal has been lost due to oversight of a seemingly minor detail.

Both contract and grant vehicles are important to the financial health of a health services or public health organization, although one vehicle or another may be a better fit at any given point in the organization's life cycle. In the application process for both of these vehicles, organizations must quickly and precisely hone in on exactly what is being asked in the application and determine if this fits within its mission, scope, and reach. Assuming that the RFP does fit the organizational scope, the organization must then garner appropriate resources to compete effectively for the funding vehicle.

Proposals may be written in response to a "request for proposal" (RFP) or to a "solicited grant announcement" (SGA). Researchers may also submit to agencies unsolicited proposals. This is like throwing a proposal over the transom. In tight economic times, unsolicited proposals have a limited chance of winning. When starting in the proposal-writing enterprise, it is common to have about a 10% win rate.

Foundation and Corporate Foundation Proposal Overview

Foundations and corporate foundations play an important philanthropic role in supporting nonprofit organizations. Gifts from foundations can represent strategic portions of an organization's overall finances, particularly for specific programs and/or projects.

- *Foundation:* an organization created from designated funds from which the income is distributed annually as grants to not-for-profit organizations, groups, and/or individuals.
- *Corporate foundation:* a private foundation funded by a profit-making corporation that has, as its primary purpose, the distribution of grants according to established guidelines.

Both foundations and corporate foundations have strict guidelines for funding areas that support their missions as well as detailed application processes. To be most successful when applying to a foundation or corporate foundation for support, the "actual components of the document include executive summary, statement of need, project description, budget, organizational information and conclusion" (Foundation Center, 2001). These components, while standard, are best when infused with impact statements, a sense of urgency, a vision, and a strong understanding of proposed project's vitality.

Many public health and health services organizations that are developing funding relationships with foundations and corporate foundations must initially be prepared to take small steps. In this competitive arena, funders often want to "try out" an organization by making a small, initial gift in order to ensure that the organization delivers on its end of the agreement: results, reports, open communication, and proper publicity. Once an organization "proves" itself, the foundation often increases its next award based on a strong second or follow-up proposal.

Individual/Family Proposal Overview

As the greatest source of philanthropy in the United States, individuals and families deserve significant attention in an organization's fundraising plan. And while the most substantial financial result is generally through a long-term relationship, there are many short- and medium-term strategies to build a strong individual/family donor base.

Figure 11–2 lists the most common fundraising approaches for soliciting individuals. While a health services or public health organization will certainly receive philanthropic support from many of these sources, it is important to understand where the potential is greatest. This diagram measures effectiveness, which often indicates the potential for the largest financial gain.

Philanthropy given by individuals is driven by each person's needs, interests, circumstances, and goals. This means that each approach is unique but grounded in the organiza-

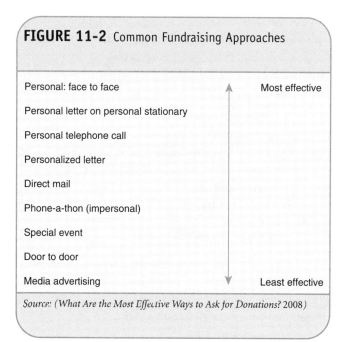

FIGURE 11-2 Common Fundraising Approaches

Personal: face to face	Most effective
Personal letter on personal stationary	
Personal telephone call	
Personalized letter	
Direct mail	
Phone-a-thon (impersonal)	
Special event	
Door to door	
Media advertising	Least effective

Source: (What Are the Most Effective Ways to Ask for Donations? 2008)

tion's mission, vision, and strategic plan. Generally, broad appeals to individuals, such as through direct mail or phone-a-thons, seek general organizational support based on the mission or a particular project/project of import. However, more significant appeals are often quite individualized and target particular interests of the individual. For example, an organization may build a relationship with a donor over time by asking for low- and mid-level gifts to support unrestricted or broadly restricted goals. However, ultimately, the public health or health services organization may ask that a particular individual create a significant fund to help pursue a particular project that is a priority for him or her and the organization.

Organizations that have the strongest philanthropic base invest significantly in fundraising programs that seek gifts from individuals through most of the methods listed earlier. These organizations focus on both current gifts as well as estate gifts. Many start-up organizations do not have the budget to support a wide-ranging individual gifts program, but they build successful programs starting with direct mail, phone-a-thons, special events, and personalized letters.

Fundraising Staffing

All members of an organization play a part in fundraising, whether they have "fundraiser" in their title or not. From the executive director to the field scientist, everyone should feel invested in and understand their role in the fundraising process. This is not to say that all staff members are equally responsible

or that everyone plays similar roles. However, in the most successful fundraising organizations, every member of the team understands how he or she helps promote a culture of philanthropy within the broad community. And fundraising activities do not need to be executed in-house to be effective. In fact, outsourcing an organization's fundraising operations, or parts of them, may be a very effective use of resources.

Fundraising staffing patterns are as unique as organizational missions. There is no one most effective staffing pattern. Organizations generally start with a small staff, sometimes even one part-time person, who focuses mainly on writing grants, creating and executing awareness events, and building a donor base of individuals through personal contact. Additional staff is added as the organization gains a better understanding of its core funding opportunities, whether that be with government grants/contracts, foundations/corporate foundations, or individuals/families.

Organizations must remember that carving out adequate budget and staffing for fundraising efforts represents bottom-line financial gain, and they must appropriate resources accordingly. In some cases, creating appropriate staffing patterns may mean reallocating parts of current positions to focus on revenue generation. Organizations cannot do part-time fundraising successfully; they must commit fully in order to gain the momentum and energy needed.

Additionally, fundraising is not simply a staff responsibility; it is also supported through a volunteer network. These volunteer partners provide essential philanthropic work for an organization. They serve as donors, governing board members, community liaisons, event hosts, network enhancers, and sounding boards. And while working with volunteers in these capacities is a significant expenditure of staff time, the payoff for an organization is important. These investments broaden the organization's base of donors and ensure the greatest opportunity for success as they expand networks to sustain and increase funding.

Staff should always be recruiting volunteers for several reasons:

Many organizations have time limits on how long volunteers can serve in the same capacity. This is to permit new blood and new ideas to enter the volunteer stream because these new members continually renew and re-energize the organization.

The recruiting activity permits the staff to be visible in a variety of communities.

As agencies change and grow, different skills sets may be required that are outside of the current volunteer-group skill set. Adding new volunteers will enable the staff to recruit for these needed new skills.

Staffing can also be maximized by building strategic partnerships with other organizations. With creative collaborations, health services and public health organizations can cultivate partners who align with and expand their mission as well as help increase the bottom line through fundraising collaborations. Over the past years, more and more fundraising dollars have supported opportunities that engage multiple organizations. Donors want to leverage their investments and partner with organizations that are doing likewise. Organizations need to invest in building collaborations because those who do not will find themselves isolated as others expand their reach and influence into new communities.

Ethics

Fundraising ethics have come to the national forefront in the last decade as several high-profile not-for-profit organizations have been publically accused of system abuses. The fundraising profession takes these charges very seriously and has actively worked to gain back lost public trust. To help safeguard an organization, health services and public health leaders and managers need to be vigilant about how they engage with fundraising prospects and donors. "Friend raising" is an apt term for defining the relationship between organization and donor. Donations cannot be made in exchange for undue influence in arenas such as choice of organizational vendors, access to organizational resources designated for others, and/or access to "classified" information. The quid pro quo relationship in fundraising is that the donor helps the organization move forward its mission and vision. The donor receives appropriate stewardship and sincere gratitude, but not unfettered access.

In fact, the Association of Fundraising Professionals (AFP) has defined ethical, professional behavior in its Code of Ethical Principals and Standards, which applies to all of its more than 30,000 members. The first tenant of the code states that "AFP members, both individual and business, aspire to practice their profession with integrity, honesty, truthfulness and adherence to the absolute obligation to safeguard the public trust" (AFP, 1964). Additionally, AFP created the Donor Bill of Rights in conjunction with the Association for Hospital Philanthropy, the Council for Advancement and Support of Education, and the Giving Institute: Leading Consultants to Non-Profits. The first tenant of the Donor Bill of Rights is that donors have the right "to be informed of the organization's mission, of the way the organization intends to use donated resources, and of its capacity to use donations effectively for their intended purposes" (AFP, *Donor Bill of Rights*).

Organizations, whether new or longstanding, must be vigilant about fundraising ethics because philanthropy occurs in the public forum. Public health and health service organizations need to have self-monitoring processes in place to focus on areas such as:

- Accounting standards.
- Organizational accountability.
- Organizational policies, including gift acceptance, investment policies, and spending policies.
- Gift agreements.
- Fee-based fundraisers.
- Donor privacy.
- Conflict of interest.

Models and prototypes of each of these processes are readily available on the Internet, as well as through professional organizations, and need to be incorporated into the standard operations manual and procedures of the agency.

Transparent Budget

Financially sound public health and health services organizations are supported by detailed, well-managed, and transparent budgets. These budgets help inform the fundraising strategic plan and provide important links in areas such as accountability, time, and accounting and fiscal responsibility. In strong organizations, fundraising and finance work closely together because as an organization's budget becomes more and more dependent on fundraising work, it is vital that there is open communication about trends, windfalls, and shortfalls.

Issues of finance and accounting can have long-standing effects on the vitality of an organization. While the Sarbanes-Oxley Act does not currently cover nonprofit agencies, it is beginning to trickle down, and it is only a matter of time before that legislation is expanded. In fact, "several state legislatures have already passed or are considering legislation containing elements of the Sarbanes-Oxley Act to be applied to nonprofit organizations… Nonprofit leaders should look carefully at the provisions of Sarbanes-Oxley, as well as their state laws, and determine whether their organizations ought to voluntarily adopt governance best practices, even if not mandated by law" (Board Source, 2003).

When determining an organization's administrative (or overhead) budget, fundraising support is an important component as it is both a revenue and a cost center. There are two metrics most commonly used to measure an organization's fundraising effectiveness. "One is the efficiency ratio, which compares how much a nonprofit spends on fulfilling its missions (known as its programs) with what it spends on overhead and fundraising. The other is the fundraising ratio, which compares fundraising costs as a percentage of contributions. The higher a nonprofit's efficiency ratio and the lower its fundraising percentage, the more comfortable donors will feel about giving money, knowing that most of it will be spent on programs" (Is Nonprofit Accounting Off Track?, 2007).

PROJECT MANAGEMENT

Strategic Project Management

Utilizing strategic project management techniques complements and undergirds both fundraising and budgeting. As a public health or health services organization's fundraising needs can be described in specifics rather than generalizations, they present a more easily understood message to potential donors. Donors want to understand why an organization is moving in a particular direction as they make investments in its future. Project management tools help donors visual the links among finances, deadlines, expected outcomes, and the gifts they give.

These tools also help the organization and the donor better understand all the possible partnerships available to help execute the organization's vision and plans. Donors and volunteers are vital links to forming creative, mutually beneficial partnerships with other not-for-profits, higher education institutions, local agencies, and for-profit entities. And while fundraising and revenue diversification can occasionally present unlikely partners, organizational leadership that is creative and open will make sound judgments about scope, organizational impact, and mission-creep juxtaposed with the ability to carry out strategic plan and mission.

Setting Organizational Strategy

Organizations that have successful fundraising programs tie fundraising strategy to the organization's strategic plan, mission, and vision. By creating this synergy and alignment, public health and health services leaders and managers lay a strong foundation for success. Once organizational priorities are aligned, fundraising goals can be created. There are three main fundraising goal components: current use priorities, capital use priorities, and endowment/long-term priorities.

To build authority for fundraising and to set actual fundraising dollar targets, health services and public health managers must consider several interrelated areas:

- *Staffing:* fundraising budget allocation and full-time-equivalent (FTE) allocation.
- *Organizational senior leadership and governance volunteers/board:* ownership of fundraising goals.

- *Program maturity:* new versus mature fundraising programs.
- *Donor readiness:* donor community understanding of fundraising goals and priorities.

If there is not alignment in these four areas before goal setting, the organization risks funding failure and the burnout of staff, volunteers, and donors.

When setting fundraising strategy, it is important to remember that there is a lag between when an organization makes an investment in fundraising and when it sees the returns. Fundraising is not a quick answer to financial hardship, but rather a strategic, long-term answer to creating organizational fortitude. Health services and public health leaders and managers of start-up organizations can reasonably expect to see fundraising results above their initial investments in a 12- to 24-month period. In some cases, this time frame may be shorter, depending on the success factors listed earlier. This time lag for new organizations demonstrates that a funding base must be built first and then enhanced. It is important to note that when the return is generated, the money is generally not given to the specific budget line that supported it, so there is not a budget offset. For example, general operating revenue might support a fundraising program, but the gifts the program seeks are for designated purposes like community outreach.

CONCLUSION

Public health and health services organizations face greater and greater competition for financial resources. Nowhere is this more evident than in the nonprofit sector. Leaders and managers need to understand the basics of fundraising so that all opportunities are brought to bear in supporting the cause and projects of the organization. Whether in a written foundation proposal or a one-on-one conversation, leaders must make their case clearly and concisely, providing financial information, project management designs, and strategic plans.

Organizations must invest critical resources to diversify funding sources and to promote a culture of philanthropy. These investments will create revenue from a variety of sources; however, the largest gains will be found by investing in long-term relationships and focusing on individuals as well as organizational donors. Government grants and contracts, as well as foundation grants, will be important parts of an organization's fundraising plan and must be factored in appropriately. And, while fundraising can seem a daunting task at times, responsibility for fundraising is not a single person's job, but rather part of everyone's job, including staff and volunteers.

Case Study

Your start-up organization's mission is to educate new mothers about the importance of vaccinating their children within the state of New York. As executive director, you have been hired by the board of directors because you have successfully run small, nonprofit organizations in the past and you have a reputation as a savvy fundraiser.

As executive director, you understand that your $500,000 start-up funding from the state ($250,000) and the Smith Family Foundation ($250,000) will cover your organization's operating expenses for the first year. The organization employs the following people: you, 1.5 FTE program managers, and a part-time office administrator. Of your initial funding, 75% is for programming. The remaining 25% must pay for staff salaries, marketing, fundraising, and overhead.

The program managers have put together project plans to support the strategic plan that launched and funded the organization initially. The board has approved both the strategic plan and the program plans. However, within these plans, additional revenue of $200,000 has been identified as needed, but no sources or plans have been presented. This shortfall includes $100,000 in both program support and overhead costs. Your board members have said that they are pleased to help with fundraising; however, no one has yet taken action.

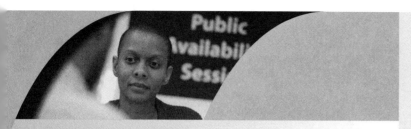

Discussion Questions

Assume you are the Executive Director.

1. Create an annual fundraising plan with a timetable, including actions and activities, as well as a staffing plan.

2. Create a revenue and expense budget for the unmet $200,000. Include a variety of funding sources, understanding that it will take more than one potential donor to meet each revenue requirement because not everyone says yes. Determine how you will pay for fundraising or if you, as executive director, will take on that significant responsibility.

3. Explain how you will motivate and utilize your board for fundraising.

4. Determine what other supporting materials you need to make the best fundraising case to potential donors.

REFERENCES

Association of Fundraising Professionals. *Code of Ethical Principals and Behaviors* adopted 1964, amended September 2007.

Association of Fundraising Professionals. *Donor Bill of Rights.*

Board Source: Building Effective Nonprofit Boards. *The Sarbanes-Oxley Act and Implications for Nonprofit Organizations.* 2003:2.

Board Source: Building Effective Nonprofit Boards: Knowledge Center. *What Are the Most Effective Ways to Ask for Donations?* 2008.

Burke RE. *Grants, Contracts, Funding Vehicles? What Are They?*: HSMP 212 presentation; April 2008.

Hrywna M. Giving USA Shows Bequests, Foundations Boosted Otherwise Flat Giving to $306 Billion. *The Nonprofit Times.* July 1, 2008.

Is Nonprofit Accounting Off Track? *Advancing Philanthropy.* September 2007:36.

The Foundation Center. *Guide to Proposal Writing.* 3rd ed; 2001:xviii.

ADDITIONAL RESOURCES

Organizations
- The Foundation Center (www.foundationcenter.org)
- Center on Philanthropy at Indiana University (www.philanthropy.iupui.edu)
- GuideStar (www.guidestar.org)
- Association of Fundraising Professionals (www.afpnet.org)
- Association for Healthcare Philanthropy (www.ahp.org)
- Counsel for the Advancement and Support of Education (www.case.org)

Publications
- *The Chronicle of Philanthropy* (www.philanthropy.com)
- *The Chronicle of Higher Education* (www.chronicle.com)

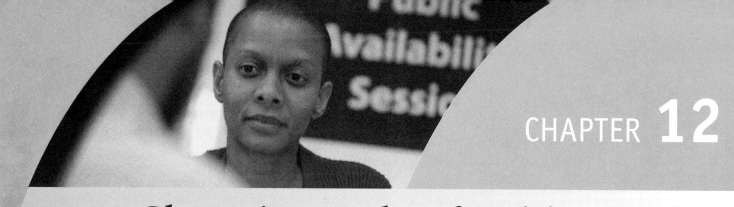

Changing Role of Public Health Managers and Leaders

Leonard H. Friedman

CHAPTER 12

Managers do things right—leaders do the right things.
—Bennis and Nanus, 1985

INTRODUCTION

One of the most interesting questions in organizations is whether there is a difference between management and leadership. This has been the topic of myriad books and articles. If you listen carefully, you will hear a consistent call for leaders in almost every sort of organization. If we can just get the right leaders with the right vision, then our public and private organizations will somehow do the right things.

Concurrent with the call for more and better leaders, people also seem to criticize those who are derisively known as "bureaucrats." Who exactly are these people, and why are they universally despised? While the term *bureaucrat* is thrown around with virtually no precision and is just a generic term for public employees at all levels, it includes persons who hold managerial or supervisory positions.

Public health organizations are dependent on both leaders and managers to do their jobs with skill, precision, and an eye on achieving the short- and long-term objectives designed to meet the needs of all stakeholder groups. As we saw earlier in this book, the lack of dependable and adequate funding needed to fulfill the many objectives of public health makes the job of management and leadership that much more challenging. The demands of stakeholders do not decrease, despite the lack of financial and personnel resources. Given this need, what are the roles of managers and leaders in public health organizations? Do these roles overlap? Can a person be both a leader and a manager, or are these jobs separate and distinct?

LEARNING OBJECTIVES

After reading this chapter, the reader will be able to:

1. Describe and distinguish the differing roles of leadership and management in healthcare organizations and predict leadership application outcomes by differentiating various leadership styles in the context of improving leadership effectiveness in the pursuit of improving public health organizations.

2. Be able to break down, compile, and regenerate leadership models, and explain, justify, and compare appropriate leadership styles in the model for healthcare contexts with the advantages and disadvantages of each.

3. Develop and justify situational-based applied leadership strategies that will improve the effectiveness of public health organizations.

4. Identify, explain, modify, and design individual leadership processes and strategies to improve public health organizations amid the dynamic healthcare environment regarding diversity, change, structural, human resources, political, and symbolic forces, and interpret possible outcomes of the leadership strategies.

LEADERSHIP PRINCIPLES

Let us begin with a short quiz. Before reading any further in this chapter, please answer the following questions based on your own personal experience and not some ideal:

- What is leadership?
- What do truly effective leaders seem to do well?
- Are there specific characteristics of persons you would consider poor leaders?
- How does leadership affect the performance of those being led?

As one point of reference, if you go to Amazon.com and search the keyword *leadership*, you will come up with more than 299,000 books where the word *leadership* appears in the title. Despite the large quantity of written material in circulation, you probably had a bit of trouble coming up with a single common definition for leadership. In lieu of coming up with a precise definition, authors have instead chosen to examine the lives of famous (or infamous) persons and looked at what it is that made them "effective" leaders. Authors have examined the leadership qualities of politicians of all stripes, military leaders, professional and collegiate athletic coaches, giants of industry, religious figures, and even 13th-century Mongol warriors. How many "leadership institutes" and consultants who specialize in leadership training are in the marketplace trying to convince you to allow them to share their secrets with you—for a price? Despite all of these examples, we continue to struggle with determining exactly what leadership means and how we can create better and more effective leaders. This is particularly important in public health organizations that generally do not have the kinds of funds to hire leaders who might be found in organizations that are better endowed financially.

For sake of discussion, let us agree (at least for the moment) on the following definition of leadership:

> Leadership is a process through which an individual attempts to intentionally influence human systems in order to accomplish a goal (Pointer, 2006).

There are a number of operational attributes of leadership that cut across all leaders, regardless of their organizations:

- "Leadership" is a process—we should consider it an action word. Leadership presumes purposeful and dynamic action on the part of the leader.
- Only individuals lead—organizations, groups, buildings, or other inanimate entities do not lead. Leadership is an intensely personal activity.
- The focus of leadership is on other individuals or groups—great leaders need great followers.
- Leadership means influencing—the question is who or what is being influenced. People have a choice about deciding to be led. The best a leader can do is successfully influence the behavior of the followers.
- The objective of leadership is goal accomplishment—the leader serves as the instrument by which organizational goals are met.
- Leadership is intentional rather than accidental—people set out to lead others. Sometimes we unintentionally influence others by what we say or do. While a good outcome, this is not leadership.
- Leadership is not confined to the executive suite.
- Leadership requires a significant degree of personal courage.

- Leadership is highly situational and is dependent on the leader, the organization, and the environment.

LEADERSHIP ROLES AND POWER

Leaders know that in order to influence people and get others to sometimes do those things that they might not otherwise do themselves, a degree of power is needed and necessary. *Power* need not be a pejorative term; without a measure of power exercised by leaders, chaos is often the result among followers. Power used in a way that is corrupt or for the achievement of goals unrelated to the mission of the organization is both highly immoral and potentially illegal. For the purposes of this chapter, we briefly discuss five forms of power commonly used by leaders to influence others (Longest, Rakich, & Darr, 2000):

- *Legitimate:* this form of power comes from one's official position in the organization. Looking at an organization chart suggests that someone has power over those below them, particularly those who are the person's direct reports.
- *Reward:* in this case, power results from the ability to reward certain behavior by pay, bonuses, promotions, gifts, etc.
- *Coercive:* leaders who exercise this type of power use their ability to punish followers for not doing what the leader wants. Examples might be demotion or termination of employment.
- *Expert:* this form of power is derived from the specific knowledge required by the organization. Often, expert power is assumed when persons have advanced academic degrees or training. Another example might be found in a person who has significant managerial or leadership experience in a similar organization.
- *Referent:* sometimes called charismatic power, these individuals create admiration, loyalty, and the desire to copy the actions of the leader among followers.

These five forms of power are complementary and should be part of the skill set of every leader. The most effective leaders know how and when to use each type of power and not to depend exclusively on one or another. Henry Mintzberg (1983) says that leadership is, "The ability to use the bases of power effectively—to convince those to whom one has access, to use one's resources, information, and technical skills to their fullest in bargaining, to exercise formal power with a sensitivity to the feelings of others, to know where to concentrate one's energies, to sense what is possible, and to organize the necessary alliances."

One of the earliest efforts to categorize leadership styles came from the work of Kurt Lewin (Lewin, Lippit, & White, 1939). This work was adopted by the U.S. Army to help prepare new officers. According to Lewin, there are three primary leadership styles: authoritative, participative, and delegative (Clark, 2004).

The *authoritative style* is used when leaders tell their employees what they want done and how they want it accomplished, without getting the advice of their followers. Some of the appropriate conditions for its use include when you have all the information necessary to solve the problem, you are short on time, and your employees are well-motivated. Some people tend to think of this style as a vehicle for yelling, using demeaning language, leading by threats, and abusing power. This is not the authoritarian style: rather, it is an abusive, unprofessional style called *bossing people around*. It has no place in a leader's repertoire. The authoritarian style should normally only be used on rare occasions. If you have the time and want to gain more commitment and motivation from your employees, then you should use the participative style.

The *participative style* involves the leader including one or more employees in the decision-making process (determining what to do and how to do it). However, the leader maintains the final decision-making authority. Using this style is not a sign of weakness, rather it is a sign of strength that your employees will respect. This is normally used when you have part of the information needed and your employees have other parts. Note that a leader is not expected to know everything—this is why you employ well-trained and prepared employees. Using this style is of mutual benefit: it allows them to become part of the team and allows you to make better decisions.

The *delegative style* allows employees to make decisions. However, the leader is still responsible for the decisions that are made. This is used when employees are able to analyze the situation and determine what needs to be done and how to do it. The leader cannot do everything! You must set priorities and delegate certain tasks. This is not a style to use so that you can blame others when things go wrong; rather, this is a style to be used when you fully trust and have confidence in the people below you.

A good leader uses all three styles, depending on what forces are involved among the followers, the leader, and the situation. Some examples include:

- Using an authoritarian style on a new employee who is just learning the job. The leader is competent and a good coach. The employee is motivated to learn a new skill, and the situation is a new environment for the employee.
- Using a participative style with a team of workers who know their job. The leader knows the problem, but does not have all the information. The employees know their jobs and want to become part of the team.
- Using a delegative style with a worker who knows more about the job than you. The employee needs to take ownership of his or her job. Also, the situation might call for you to be at other places, doing other things.

- Using all three. For example, telling your employees that a procedure is not working correctly and a new one must be established (authoritarian); asking for their ideas and input on creating a new procedure (participative); assigning tasks in order to implement the new procedure (delegative) (Clark, 2004).

THEORIES OF LEADERSHIP

Leaders have been part of social systems since humans first walked the face of the earth. In primitive societies, it was the strongest or wisest person who was the leader of the tribe or clan. In ancient Greece, there were writings about the need for leaders to emerge as part of their political system. In the early 20th century, we began to see significant attention paid to leadership and what it was that leaders had in common with one another. It is from this literature that three schools of thought began to emerge: the trait, behavior, and contingency theories of leadership.

Trait Perspective

Early in the study of leaders and leadership, people wondered if there were "born" leaders: that is, persons who just knew how to lead others without any formal training or education. The early work on leadership traits concentrated on military commanders and those who held political office. There have literally been thousands of studies, and the traits that seem to be commonly found among leaders are intelligence, articulateness, confidence, initiative, persistence, and sociability (Pointer, 2006).

If traits were the things that mattered most in leaders, then it would be easy to identify persons who displayed those attributes—particularly if they could be found early. We know that there is no standard set of traits that equate to leadership. There are a number of other potential downsides to the trait perspective. Traits can influence personal behavior that activates leadership. They are a necessary but not sufficient condition. You cannot separate out a single trait (or group of traits) and claim that it alone causes leadership. Finally, as stated earlier, leadership is a function of the behavior of the leader and not simply the collection of specific traits.

Behavior Perspective

Researchers have long searched for those particular behaviors that were characteristic of the most effective leaders with the idea of developing models for leadership styles. Some of the earliest research into the behavioral perspective on leadership was done in the first part of the 20th century by Kurt Lewin and his colleagues at the University of Iowa. He categorized leadership behavior as autocratic, democratic, or laissez-faire. The *autocratic* leaders made decisions without the input of the members of the group whereas *democratic* leaders sought to make decisions on the basis the rule of the majority. The *laissez-faire* leaders provided neither direction to group members nor interaction with the group. They just let things occur.

One of the most well-known studies was done at The Ohio State University in the years just after World War II (Stodgill & Coons, 1957). In this case, a questionnaire was handed out to industrial and military employees to measure their perceptions of the leaders in each industry and the behavior of these leaders. This research came out with two dimensions of behavior:

- *Consideration:* a highly considerate leader who is sensitive to people's feelings and tries to make things pleasant for the followers.
- *Initiating structure:* a kind of leader who is concerned with spelling out the task requirement and clarifying other aspects of the work agenda.

These two dimensions were researched more intensely by scholars, including Fleischman, 1973, Korman, 1966 and Likert 1961, to discover which leadership style is the best. The conclusion of this study was that leaders need to have both consideration and initiating structure to be a successful leader.

One of the particularly interesting and important studies was done by Blake and Mouton (1978), who synthesized the work of several other researchers to develop their well-known managerial grid. As you can see in **Figure 12-1**, the grid is set

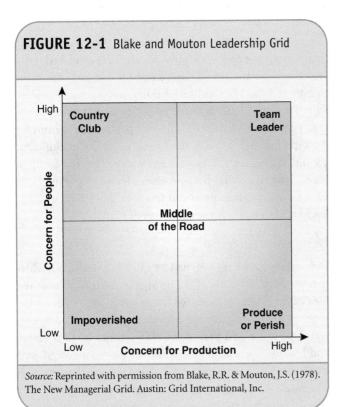

FIGURE 12-1 Blake and Mouton Leadership Grid

Source: Reprinted with permission from Blake, R.R. & Mouton, J.S. (1978). The New Managerial Grid. Austin: Grid International, Inc.

up along two dimensions, production and people. When using a *production* focus, leader behaviors are directed on accomplishing assigned objectives and tasks. When focused on *people*, the behavior of the leader is centered on enhancing the quality of manager–follower and follower–follower interactions. The behavior of the leader can range from low to high on both dimensions, which according to Blake and Mouton, results in five possible leadership styles.

Produce or Perish Leader (High Production, Low People)

Leaders who get this rating are very much task oriented and are hard on their workers (autocratic). There is little or no allowance for cooperation or collaboration. Heavily task-oriented people display the following characteristics: they are very strong on schedules; they expect people to do what they are told without question or debate; when something goes wrong, they tend to focus on who is to blame rather than concentrate on exactly what is wrong and how to prevent it; and they are intolerant of what they see as dissent (it may just be someone's creativity), so it is difficult for their subordinates to contribute or develop.

Team Leader (High Production, High People)

These persons lead by positive example and endeavor to foster a team environment in which all team members can reach their highest potential, both as team members and as people. They encourage the team to reach team goals as effectively as possible, while also working tirelessly to strengthen the bonds among the various members. They normally form and lead some of the most productive teams.

Country Club Leader (Low Production, High People)

These persons predominantly use reward power to maintain discipline and to encourage the team to accomplish its goals. Conversely, they are almost incapable of employing the more punitive coercive and legitimate powers. This inability results from fear that using such powers could jeopardize relationships with the other team members.

Impoverished Leader (Low Production, Low People)

These leaders use a "delegate and disappear" management style. Because they are not committed to either task accomplishment or maintenance, they essentially allow their team to do whatever it wishes and prefer to detach themselves from the team process by allowing the team to suffer from a series of power struggles.

Middle-of-the-Road Leader (Moderate Production, Moderate People)

Leaders who use this style are able to balance goal and task accomplishment in addition to need fulfillment of followers.

Contingency Perspectives

Despite the best efforts of researchers and consultants alike, trying to make sense of leadership from exclusively a trait or behavior perspective proved to be a futile exercise. Perhaps the answer to defining great leadership was a combination of both perspectives into something that came to be called the *contingency model*. One of the first contingency models was developed by Tannenbaum and Schmidt (1973), as pictured in **Figure 12-2**.

In this model, leadership behavior is viewed as a continuum ranging from boss- (leader) centered to subordinate-centered. As you can easily see, the person in charge has a wide range of options available, depending on the situation at hand. In a crisis, it makes sense for the leader to make and announce his or her decision as opposed to obtaining group buy-in. When the leader has the luxury of time, a more subordinate-centered form of leadership style is in order. It should be clear that there is no single leadership style equally effective in all situations. It is also important to consider the characteristics of the leader, the followers, and the environment in which the people interact.

A second important contingency model is the *leadership match model*, originally developed by Fred Fiedler (1967). His idea was that managers are unable to change their leadership style to any appreciable degree. Leadership effectiveness is dependent on selecting a situation that is the best fit for a person's style. A classic example of matching the leadership style with the situation is the case of Mayor Rudolph Guliani of New York. Prior to September 11, 2001, he was widely regarded as (at best) an average leader who held little influence in his city, despite his formal leadership role and title. By all accounts, the events of 9/11 showed Mayor Guliani to be extremely effective in a crisis environment. He was the same person both before and after the events of that day, but his leadership style was a much better match for the chaos and rapid decisions that needed to be made when New York needed a truly decisive mayor.

The *path-goal contingency model* of leadership (Vroom, 1964) is based on the expectancy theory of motivation. That is, people are motivated to do things when they expect some sort of reward for their efforts. The reward can take many forms and includes things such as salary, bonuses, recognition, advancement, or another form of tangible payoff. The role of the leader is to align his or her leadership style with the availability of rewards that are most meaningful to the followers.

The final contingency model discussed here is termed *attribution theory*. In this case, the selection of a particular leadership style by the manager is driven by the way follower

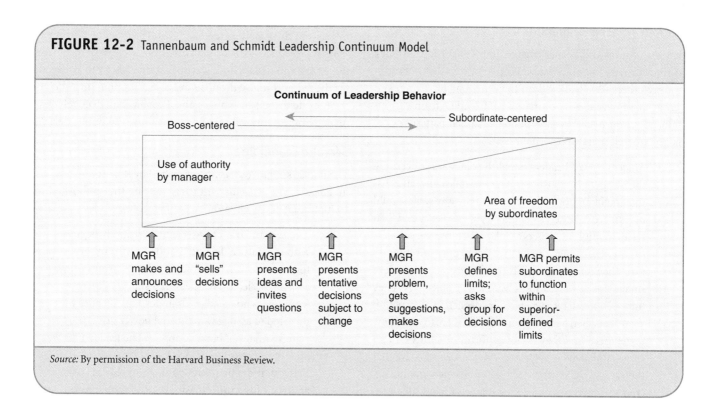

FIGURE 12-2 Tannenbaum and Schmidt Leadership Continuum Model

Source: By permission of the Harvard Business Review.

behavior is perceived and interpreted (Mitchell, Green, & Wood, 1981). Managers notice some things and are unaware of others. Those things that are noticed are filtered and viewed through the manager's personal frame of reference. Based on the managers' perceptions, followers tend to behave in certain ways. In the same way, managers perceive their employees in certain ways and they behave accordingly. For example, leadership behavior will be significantly different if the manager believes that the subordinate is lazy as opposed to being poorly trained to do a certain task. In a community health department, a leader might excuse an employee's chronic tardiness to the fact that the employee has child care issues or personal health concerns as opposed to a framework that the person cannot seem to get out of bed and get to work on time.

ALTERNATIVE LEADERSHIP PERSPECTIVES

In addition to the well-known and highly respected thoughts on leadership previously mentioned, there are a number of more contemporary perspectives that persons in public health organizations will likely find appealing. The alternative perspectives that are part of this discussion include evidence-based leadership, servant leadership, transformational leadership, and emotional intelligence and leadership. It is likely that public health professionals will be drawn to these alternative perspectives given the highly mission-focused activities of their organizations, coupled with the strong service orientation found in the vast majority of public health settings.

Evidence-Based Leadership

In 1983, Kouzes and Posner began a four-year study designed to find out what people did when they were at their best in leading others (2007). Based on their analysis of written and verbal surveys done with more than 550 leaders from various industries, Kouzes and Posner found five similar patterns of behavior when leaders were at their best:

- *Model the way.* Leaders establish principles concerning the way people (constituents, peers, colleagues, and customers alike) should be treated and the way goals should be pursued. They create standards of excellence and then set an example for others to follow. Because the prospect of complex change can overwhelm people and stifle action, they set interim goals so that people can achieve small wins as they work toward larger objectives. They unravel bureaucracy when it impedes action, they put up signposts when people are unsure of where to go or how to get there, and they create opportunities for victory.
- *Inspire a shared vision.* Leaders passionately believe that they can make a difference. They envision the future, creating an ideal and unique image of what the organization can become. Through their magnetism and quiet persuasion, leaders enlist others in their dreams. They breathe life into their visions and get people to see exciting possibilities for the future.
- *Challenge the process.* Leaders search for opportunities to change the status quo. They look for innovative ways to improve the organization. In doing so, they experiment and take risks. And because leaders know that risk taking involves mistakes and failures, they accept the inevitable disappointments as learning opportunities.
- *Enable others to act.* Leaders foster collaboration and build spirited teams. They actively involve others. Leaders understand that mutual respect is what sustains extraordinary efforts; they strive to create an atmosphere of trust and human dignity. They strengthen others, making each person feel capable and powerful.
- *Encourage the heart.* Accomplishing extraordinary things in organizations is hard work. To keep hope and determination alive, leaders recognize contributions that individuals make. In every winning team, the members need to share in the rewards of their efforts, so leaders celebrate accomplishments. They make people feel like heroes.

The Kouzes and Posner framework is most applicable for persons in public health. The idea of creating a shared vision as a rallying point for all staff members is crucial given the fact that most public health organizations are highly mission-centered. For example, most (if not all) public health organizations are chronically understaffed and frequently cannot pay market-based salaries for staff members. Leaders recognize these facts and need to find ways other than salary to keep staff motivated and focused on the mission. Tapping into the attributes described by Kouzes and Posner can effectively resonate with the core values of persons drawn to public health.

Servant Leadership

The phrase *servant leadership* was coined by Robert K. Greenleaf in *The Servant as Leader*, an essay that he first published in 1970. In that essay, he said:

> The servant-leader *is* servant first . . . It begins with the natural feeling that one wants to serve, to serve *first.* Then conscious choice brings one to aspire to lead. That person is sharply different from one who is *leader* first, perhaps because of the need to assuage an unusual power drive or to acquire material possessions . . . The leader-first and the servant-first are two extreme types. Between them there are shadings and blends that are part of the infinite variety of human nature.

The difference manifests itself in the care taken by the servant-first to make sure that other people's highest priority needs are being served. The best test, and difficult to administer, is: Do those served grow as persons? Do they, *while being served*, become healthier, wiser, freer, more autonomous, more likely themselves to become servants? *And*, what is the effect on the least privileged in society? Will they benefit or at least not be further deprived?

There are a number of important attributes of servant leaders:

- Listening receptively to what others have to say.
- Acceptance of others and having empathy for them.
- Foresight and intuition.
- Awareness and perception.
- Highly developed powers of persuasion.
- Ability to conceptualize and to communicate those ideas.
- Ability to exert a healing influence upon individuals and institutions.
- Building community in the workplace.
- Practicing the art of contemplation.
- Recognition that servant leadership begins with the desire to change oneself.

As was the case with evidence-based leadership, servant leadership is a framework that should be very appealing to public health organizations. Pay attention to the language used by Greenleaf. In this model, the leader is most concerned with the welfare of the members of the organization and leadership exists to meet the employees' needs first.

Transformational Leadership

Developed initially for political leaders by James McGregor Burns in the late 1970s, *transformational leadership* was eagerly adopted for business leadership. It has four components: charisma or idealized influence, inspirational motivation, intellectual stimulation, and individualized consideration. Being charismatic involves possessing a dynamic, energetic, and commanding presence. We idealize such people. Robert F. Kennedy is a great example of a transformational leader. Leaders who are inspirational motivators appeal to basic values with enthusiasm and an eloquent speaking style to offer a compelling vision. Intellectual stimulation means inspiring people to think differently or creatively by suggesting new ways of looking at things. Finally, showing individualized consideration means paying attention to people as individuals and helping them meet their needs. Burns and his followers contrasted transformational leadership with *transactional leadership*, which is based on sim-

ple exchange, or rewarding followers for a job well done (McCrimmon, 2008).

Most leadership models are said to be transactional. Think about the path-goal model discussed earlier in this chapter. The leader determines the particular goal that needs to be accomplished and then works to activate the right kind of motivation for each staff member in order to help achieve that goal. If the staff member does what is asked, the anticipated reward will be provided. Transactional leadership is based on maintaining the status quo and requires that members make sure to play by the rules. Transformational leadership works to upset the status quo and, rather than playing by the rules, requires that leaders intentionally work to break the rules.

Emotional Intelligence and Leadership

In 1995, Daniel Goleman published what proved to be one of the most important current books on leadership when he popularized the idea of *emotional intelligence*. He described four core competencies that help to enhance leadership performance:

- *Self-awareness:* the ability to read one's emotions and recognize their impact while using gut feelings to guide decisions.
- *Self-management:* involves controlling one's emotions and impulses and adapting to changing circumstances.
- *Social awareness:* the ability to sense, understand, and react to others' emotions while comprehending social networks.
- *Relationship management:* the ability to inspire, influence, and develop others while managing conflict.

If you think about your own experience in the workplace, you realize that it is impossible to separate people from their emotions. We are, at our core, emotional beings. Perhaps one of the smartest things that public health leaders can do is to acknowledge and work with their own emotions and those of the people throughout their organization.

CONCLUSION

Effective and visionary leadership is particularly critical in public health organizations for a number of important reasons. A combination of a strong mission, scarce resources, and a need to serve a broad community of stakeholders makes leadership an absolute necessity. This chapter has shown us that leadership is an activity that requires more than just thought and contemplation. At its core, leadership requires action. Persons who assume leadership roles must possess a high level of courage. You will be asked to take your organization and staff in directions that will challenge everyone to envision their work and provision of services to clients in new and different ways. One of the things we hope you take from this chapter is that leadership is not reserved just for persons in senior management positions. People throughout the organization can be leaders regardless of title—or lack thereof. While it is possible to learn and practice certain skills that seem to be common to leaders, there are also a number of traits that must be part of who you are. The question is how that combination of skills and traits is put to best use and under what circumstances. We have examined a number of important theories about leadership and have seen that there is no one right answer. Leadership is highly situational and is dependent on both the individual leader and the organizational environment that is in place. We know that persons who are effective leaders in one environment need not be equally effective in another and, in fact, might be an abject failure. We have seen that many of the contemporary perspectives on leadership make clear that we must attend to the hearts and minds of our followers—simply putting out the right rewards and motivating people to do certain things has a place, but it is not sufficient for leaders in public health settings. We must pay attention to the emotional core of both ourselves and those we want to lead. Simply put, leadership is a complex set of behaviors that must acknowledge our own skills and traits as well as those of the persons being led. There is no one perfect model of leadership. Rather, there are multiple models—all of which have their place, depending on the demands of the organization and the environment in which it operates.

CLOSING THOUGHTS AND FURTHER READINGS

Public health organizations require both outstanding management and visionary leadership. One of the most succinct and readable books on leadership was written in 1986 by Warren Bennis and Burt Nanus. Their research shows us that truly effective leaders continually do four things particularly well:

- Provide attention through vision.
- Provide meaning through communication.
- Provide trust through positioning.
- Provide deployment of self through positive self-regard.

Creation of a vision is about the clear focus on a particular long-term goal. This is the "North Star" or the rallying point that others in the organization can see as the outcome they wish to achieve. In the words of the authors, "vision is the target that beckons." The most effective leaders find a way to continually communicate that vision, which helps create and sustain people even when they become discouraged. Trust is the emotional glue of the organization. Leaders cannot achieve organizational goals by themselves. They need the ongoing efforts of staff and must trust their staff to move toward desired goals. Trust must be earned—it is never conferred. Finally, leaders must believe in themselves and, at the same time, must be open to new ideas and continual learning. The best leaders have a high level of self-awareness and understand their emotional makeup and how they affect the work of others.

There is no question that scholars and practitioners will continue to research, write, think, argue, and debate about leadership. Your task in this highly uncertain and confusing time is to go beyond reading about leadership and instead do those things that you wish to see in the very best leaders. The journey will never be easy, but your organization and the people you serve depend on you to demonstrate your willingness to become the person that others will follow.

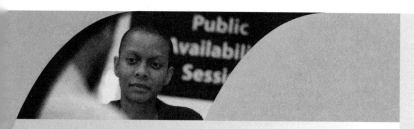

Discussion Questions

1. Under what circumstances would it make sense for a public health leader to adopt an authoritarian style?

2. You often hear that leaders are born and not made. At the same time, you read about leadership training programs of all sorts. How can you reconcile the difference? Are there people who are born leaders? Can you learn how to become a leader?

3. Where do you think you fall on the Blake and Mouton leadership grid? Do you think that your leadership style has changed over time?

4. How well do you think that an evidence-based leadership perspective, such as the one put forward by Kouzes and Posner, works in a public health setting?

5. Distinguish between transactional and transformational leadership. How might each one be used in a public health organization?

REFERENCES

Bennis W, Nanus B. *Leaders: Strategies for Taking Charge.* New York: Harper and Row; 1985.

Blake RR, Mouton JS. *The New Managerial Grid.* Houston, TX: Gulf Publishing Company; 1978.

Burns JM. *Leadership.* New York: McGraw-Hill; 1978.

Clark DR. Instructional System Design Concept Map. *Leadership Styles.* Available at: http://nwlink.com/~donclark/hrd/ahold/isd.html. Accessed October 24, 2008.

Fiedler FE. *A Theory of Leadership Effectiveness.* New York: McGraw-Hill; 1967.

Fleishman FA. Twenty years of consideration and structure. In: Fleishman FA, Hunts JG, eds. *Current developments in the study of leadership.* Carbondale, IL: Southern Illinois University; 1973:1–37.

Goleman D. *Emotional Intelligence.* New York: Bantam Books; 1995.

Greenleaf RK. *The Servant as Leader.* Personal Essay.

Korman AK. Consideration, initiating structure and organizational criteria: a review. *Personnel Psychology.* 1966;19:349–361.

Kouzes JM, Posner BZ. *The Leadership Challenge.* 4th ed. San Francisco: Jossey-Bass; 2007.

Lewin K, Lippitt R, White RK. Patterns of aggressive behavior in experimentally created social climates. *Journal of Social Psychology.* 1939;10:271–301.

Likert R. *New patterns of management.* New York: McGraw-Hill; 1961.

Longest BB, Rakich JS, Darr K. *Managing Health Services Organizations and Systems.* Chicago: Health Professions Press; 2000.

McCrimmon M. *Transformational Leadership: Benefits & limitations of transformational leadership.* Business Management. Available at: http://businessmanagement.suite101.com/article.cfm/transformational_leadership. Accessed February 18, 2010.

Mintzberg H. *Power in and Around Organizations (The Theory of Management Policy).* Englewood Cliffs, NJ: Prentice Hall; 1983.

Mitchell TR, Green SG, Wood RE. An attributional model of leadership and the poor performing subordinate: Development and Validation. In: Staw B, Cummings LL, eds. *Research in Organizational Behavior.* Stamford, CT: JAI Press; 1981.

Pointer DD. Leadership: A framework for thinking and acting. In: Shortell SM, Kalunzy AD, eds. *Health Care Management.* Clifton Park, NY: Delmar Publishers; 2006.

Stodgill, RM, Coons AE. (Eds). Leader behavior: Its description and measurement. A research monograph, No. 88. *Bureau of Business Research,* The Ohio State University, Columbus, Ohio: 1957.

Tannenbaum R, Schmidt WH. How to choose a leadership pattern. *Harvard Business Review.* 1973;51:162–180.

Vroom VH. Work and motivation. In: Wagner JA, Hollenback JR, eds. *Management of Organizational Behavior.* Englewood Cliffs, NJ: Prentice Hall; 1964.

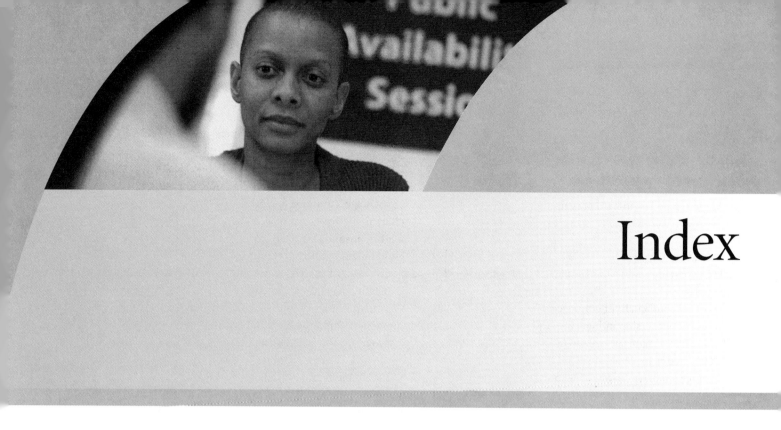

Index